T0132181

THE LONGEVITY PRESCRIPTION

ALSO BY ROBERT N. BUTLER

AUTHOR

Human Aging (with J. E. Birren, S. W. Greenhouse, L. Sokoloff, and M. R. Yarrow)

Aging and Mental Health (with M. I. Lewis; 5th edition with T. Sunderland)

Why Survive? Being Old in America

Love and Sex After Sixty (with M. I. Lewis)

EDITOR

The Aging Process (with A. G. Bearn)

Productive Aging: Enhancing Vitality in Later Life (with H. P. Gleason)

Aging in Liver and Gastrointestinal Tract
(with L. Bianchi, P. Holt, O.F.W. James, and L. Landmann)

Human Aging Research (with B. Kent)

Modern Biological Theories of Aging (with H. R. Warner, E. Schneider, and R. L. Sprott)

The Promise of Productive Aging (with M. Oberlink and M. Schechter)

Who Is Responsible for My Old Age? (with K. Kiikuni)

Delaying the Onset of Late-Life Dysfunction (with J. A. Brody)

Cognitive Decline: Strategies for Prevention (with H. M. Fillit)

Life in an Older America (with L. K. Grossman and M. R. Oberlink)

Longevity and Quality of Life (with C. Jasmin)

THE LONGEVITY PRESCRIPTION

THE 8 PROVEN KEYS TO A LONG, HEALTHY LIFE

❖

ROBERT N. BUTLER, M.D.

PRESIDENT AND CEO
The International Longevity Center–USA

AVERY
a member of Penguin Group (USA) Inc.
New York

Published by the Penguin Group
Penguin Group (USA) Inc., 375 Hudson Street, New York, New York 10014, USA ·
Penguin Group (Canada), 90 Eglinton Avenue East, Suite 700, Toronto, Ontario M4P 2Y3,
Canada (a division of Pearson Penguin Canada Inc.) · Penguin Books Ltd, 80 Strand,
London WC2R 0RL, England · Penguin Ireland, 25 St Stephen's Green, Dublin 2, Ireland
(a division of Penguin Books Ltd) · Penguin Group (Australia), 250 Camberwell Road,
Camberwell, Victoria 3124, Australia (a division of Pearson Australia Group Pty Ltd) ·
Penguin Books India Pvt Ltd, 11 Community Centre, Panchsheel Park, New Delhi–110 017,
India · Penguin Group (NZ), 67 Apollo Drive, Rosedale, North Shore 0632, New Zealand
(a division of Pearson New Zealand Ltd) · Penguin Books (South Africa) (Pty) Ltd,
24 Sturdee Avenue, Rosebank, Johannesburg 2196, South Africa

Penguin Books Ltd, Registered Offices: 80 Strand, London WC2R 0RL, England

First trade paperback edition 2011
Copyright © 2010 by Robert N. Butler, M.D.

The Library of Congress has catalogued the hardcover edition as follows:

Butler, Robert N., date.
The longevity prescription: the 8 proven keys to a long, healthy life /
Robert N. Butler.
p.   cm.
Includes index.
ISBN 978-1-58333-388-4
1. Longevity—Popular works.   2. Longevity—Physiological aspects.
3. Aging—Prevention.   4. Health.   I. Title.
RA776.75.B88   2010   2009052682
612.6'8—dc22

ISBN 978-1-58333-430-0 (paperback edition)

BOOK DESIGN BY TANYA MAIBORODA

TO THE FAMILIES

OF

AMERICA

CONTENTS

ABOUT THE INTERNATIONAL
LONGEVITY CENTER

❄

THE INTERNATIONAL LONGEVITY CENTER–USA IS A POLICY research center concerned with population aging and longevity. Its work centers on understanding and promoting healthy aging, productive engagement, and the economics of aging, as well as quality of life issues, notably combating ageism. The center, founded in 1990 by Dr. Robert Butler at Mount Sinai Medical School, is international in scope, working in concert with sister centers around the world, and interdisciplinary, drawing on such disciplines and professional fields as medicine, health policy, economics, demographics, public health, and communications. It is now part of Columbia University. It is also intergenerational in its orientation, arguing that aging is about everyone, not just older people. Guided by a distinguished board of directors that includes two Nobel laureates and members from business, academe, law, public affairs, and philanthropy, the nonpartisan

ILC also draws on an eminent board of advisers called the Program Advisory Group and several other expert panels that provide a longevity network, which includes many national and international experts in and among the several fields that the center monitors, studies, and organizes projects around.

The center's main activities include its respected scientific consensus workshops, which have taken up such topics as healthy aging, cognitive vitality, sleep and healthy aging, and sexuality, each drawing world-class experts to a working seminar that "downloads" the best available information, integrating it into consensus reports that are widely distributed and cited. Some then become articles in peer-reviewed scientific journals, while others are less technical and go to health experts, policy makers, and members of the general public.

The center's work extends around the world through the aforementioned ILCs in the United Kingdom, France, the Netherlands, South Africa, Japan, Israel, Argentina, the Dominican Republic, the Czech Republic, India, and Singapore. It is also expressed in its acclaimed World Cities Project (New York, London, Paris, and Tokyo), a collaboration with scholars at New York University and the State University of New York. In addition, the ILC has collaborated with its UK and French partners to create the Alliance for Health and the Future, a ten-nation health policy program that has pioneered work on health and wealth as well as a series of healthy-aging Life Guides that offer advice across the generations to promote good health and longevity. Another major effort at the ILC is its Caregiving Project for Older Americans, a multiyear effort to improve the quality of caregiving education and caregiving. This project is in collaboration with the Schmieding Foundation and Schmieding Center for Senior Health and Education and involves several foundations and corporate sponsors.

For more than a decade the ILC has conducted an annual Age Boom Academy, a high-level training program for journalists and communicators concerned with aging and population issues. It also has a communications program of public outreach, publications, and a lively Web 2.0 site.

The ILC's leadership issues policy briefs and regularly testifies in Congress and before important boards, commissions, and other efforts, including the White House Conference on Aging. The ILC has special consultative status at the United Nations and is a fully accredited NGO (nongovernmental organization). In its role the ILC has provided leadership at the World Assembly on Ageing.

The ILC works closely with businesses, institutions of higher learning, government agencies, and other entities to advance the cause of longevity, healthy aging, and productive engagement.

The ILC welcomes inquiries at www.ilcusa.org.

INTRODUCTION

EMBRACING
LONGEVITY

A LONG LIFE IS A DEEP HUMAN YEARNING, ONE THAT IS AS OLD as the first gray hair. Yet the desire is not quite as simple as that. As expressed by the eighteenth-century satirist and author of *Gulliver's Travels*, Jonathan Swift, "Every man desires to live long; but no man would be old."

The aim of this book, then, is twofold: to use the accumulated knowledge, research, and resources of the International Longevity Center (ILC) in order to offer you the best strategies to live long *and* to live well.

The ILC and *The Longevity Prescription* exist for one very important reason—namely, the unprecedented increase in longevity. The average American in the year 1900 lived to age fifty. In the hundred-plus years since, life expectancy in the United States has risen dramatically to seventy-seven-plus years. In round numbers, we can anticipate living *ten thousand days* longer than our ancestors could a century ago. That's what I call the three-decade

I

dividend. The ILC's goal is to help people—that includes you—to live happier, healthier, and more productive lives during the aging years.

The average American simply does not need to resign himself or herself to spending these added decades descending slowly and unhappily into disease and disability. Aging does not have to be full of sickness and infirmity. On the contrary, there is an immense body of research that demonstrates that most of our bonus days can be lived in robust good health, both mental and physical, and in that spirit this book is dedicated to helping you feel, think, and remain younger.

That is not a dream.

You have doubts? I ask you to ponder this:

HOW IMPORTANT IS GENETIC INHERITANCE? Folk wisdom has long told us that genes determine life expectancy. That is, if your grandparents lived long, healthy lives, you can feel confident that you will, too. Conversely, you may worry that short-lived ancestors predetermine how long you will live.

More recent research, however, has found that the role your genetic inheritance plays in longevity probably is much less than you think.

Certain physical traits are clearly inherited. For example, the correlation between a child's eventual height and his parent's is between 80 and 90 percent; in the same way, genes probably get the blame for roughly two-thirds of an individual's risk of being obese. But longevity is a different matter. Even identical twins, despite sharing the same genetic inheritance, often have quite different life expectancies, typically dying ten or more years apart.

In a major study at the Institute of Gerontology at the University College of Health Sciences in Jönköping, Sweden, researchers analyzed data based on a sample of more than ten thousand sets of twins (roughly one-third identical, the balance fraternal). Some of these twins were separated at birth so the impact of nurture and nature could be compared. A detailed analysis of these data found that only about *one-third* of the variations in longevity could be attributed to genetic factors, while individual environmental factors accounted for the rest of the differences.

Such observations have led researchers to conclude that the longevity correlation between parent and child is surprisingly small. The numbers vary from study to study, but studies have consistently found a small link of between 5 and 35 percent.

In short? *Your genes do not predetermine your longevity.*

YOU ARE NOT TOO OLD TO STAY YOUNG. If you are in your fifties, sixties, or even seventy-something or beyond, there are strategies you can employ to retain—and even regain—good health.

There is clear evidence that healthy strategies can play a role in reducing the risks of osteoporosis, heart disease, hypertension, and cancer. By staying physically active, eating well, and controlling your weight, you can help avoid diabetes, the loss of mobility, and even cognitive decline. There are means of recovering lost strength, balance, and mental vitality, too.

People who live healthier lifestyles not only live longer. They also have a lower incidence of many chronic diseases and, further, the age of disease onset has been found to be three to five years later. Well into the aging years, sensible behaviors can increase your odds of living a longer and healthier life.

The message? *No matter what your age, there are ways to enhance your longevity.*

living longer

We *are* making progress.

- Archaeological findings suggest that four out of five of our prehistoric ancestors were dead by age thirty; only about one in twenty lived to age forty.
- A citizen of the Roman Empire had a life expectancy of about twenty-eight years.
- By the turn of the nineteenth century, a person in one of the more advanced countries might anticipate some thirty-five years of life.

- In the early years of the twentieth century, the average American could expect to live to about age fifty.
- Today, from the ancient Roman average of twenty-eight years, we have gain a full *fifty years* to reach our nearly seventy-eight-year life expectancy.

YOU ARE NOT TOO YOUNG TO PLAN FOR AGING. To judge by one recent long-term study, it is never too soon to consider longevity. Researchers have found a high correlation between elevated cholesterol levels in children and high serum cholesterol in the adults they had become almost thirty years later. In adults in midlife, similar patterns have also been observed.

The lesson? Bad habits are best broken early to reduce the long-term impact of high blood pressure, high cholesterol, and other health hazards. *Good habits can translate into longevity—and disease-free, healthy, productive living.*

CAN I REVERSE THE AGING PROCESS? Your cells, your bodily systems, and your mental and physical abilities will decline over a period of years; aging cannot be put on hold indefinitely. That's the reason that most professional athletes retire by age forty, and why most of us, athletic or not, begin to experience blurred vision when looking at small print in our forties. It is the explanation for those wrinkles that begin to appear around the eyes, on the neck, and elsewhere. The function of the kidneys, heart, and lungs gradually decrease with age, as does immune function. All these are entirely normal consequences of passing years.

But you can resist the tides of time. Just as conditioning regimes extend athletic careers, corrective lenses keep us reading the small print, and a blend of creams and plastic surgeries can cover or even smooth out the wrinkling, various strategies *can* address many of these changes. How we live determines a great deal about the pace at which we age. To cite just one example, healthy behaviors can reduce the level of sugars and fats in the blood and control blood pressure, all of which are risk factors for a range of age-related disorders. Studies consistently show direct health benefits (decreased incidence of stroke and heart attack) from managing hypertension.

The takeaway message? *More than a little of your long-term health is very much up to you.*

WHAT IS AGING, ANYWAY? Aging *is not* simply a matter of time. We all know people who are "old" in a chronological sense (in their eighties or nineties, perhaps) but who are clearly "young" judging by the healthy, active, and engaged manner in which they conduct their lives. Conversely, we all know "young" people (in this context, let's regard young as forty- or fifty-something) who look and act much older than they are.

To a surprising degree, aging is a state of mind. People who take a preventive approach to their health tend to stay young. By heeding warning signs like high blood pressure, weight gain, and elevated blood sugar and by making lifestyle changes, we can avoid or at least minimize some chronic diseases.

A Harris Poll not so long ago asked what the best marker of old age was. Almost no one relied upon age (just 14 percent regarded chronological age as the key indicator). It is about your health, about how you feel; the way you live and your attitude to aging can change and slow the course of aging.

Understand that the classic description of aging—*the human body is like a machine that wears out over time*—draws a false comparison. To call it a machine does not do the human anatomy justice, because the body is vastly more complicated than any mechanical device, consisting of a diverse array of systems that perform many distinct functions.

Bodily systems are interdependent, with built-in backups that enable the system as a whole to continue—that is, for life to continue—even when one or more systems fails. We have extra organs (a second lung, an extra kidney). The body's redundancies and its ability to repair itself help us carry on in the face of injury, illness, and aging.

Evidence is accruing almost daily of the ways in which the human body can regain lost functions. The risk of heart disease falls for the smoker who quits, whatever his age or the number of smoking years. Lost balance, strength, and mental vitality can be restored. It is important to see aging as a complex set of processes, some of which you can affect to enhance your health and your life.

While aging is inevitable, your decision to live well can play a crucial role in aging well.

Compression of Morbidity

You do not have to be a doctor to understand the longevity prescription, but the power and effectiveness of the strategies in this book are based on solid research. That means certain key scientific notions merit explanation. Understanding some of the science—be it medical, epidemiological, or chemical—will help you better appreciate the *whys* as well as the *hows*.

The most essential term is *compression of morbidity*. This umbrella concept was the brainchild of a pioneer in the study of aging, James F. Fries, M.D., professor of medicine at Stanford University School of Medicine. As he himself explained it, "The goal is to delay the onset of chronic illness, that kind of illness that causes most of the misery in life, to as late in life as possible."

In your middle years, chronic illness tends to be a far greater concern than death. We worry about the maladies that erode quality of life, hobble the body, sap our energy, addle our thinking, or even threaten us with relocation to a nursing home.

What we fear from aging is a period of *morbidity* (sickness) that is prolonged and progressive.

On this front, I see very good news indeed. Investigators—demographers, economists, physicians, and biological anthropologists—have assembled immense data sets that enable them to compare and contrast the health of Americans in the past to the present. To cite just one example, a study funded by the National Institute on Aging collected a vast array of information about some 45,000 veterans of the Civil War. Of the many findings that emerged from the analysis of this data, one is of particular interest to those of us who are aging in our time.

Conventional wisdom has long held that, as life expectancy increased during the twentieth century, more people spent more of those dividend years plagued by debilitating chronic illnesses. In fact, researchers have found that common ailments like heart disease, arthritis, and lung problems arrived on average a full ten years later at the turn of the twenty-first century compared to a hundred years earlier. Similarly, two and half times as many modern men entered their sixties without chronic conditions.

The explanations for this are many, but research on several fronts suggests that each of us has the power to increase our chances of remaining healthy longer, of delaying the period of decline that precedes the end of one's life. That's what doctors call compression of morbidity. You can achieve this on your own by taking some simple proactive precautions.

As we began thinking about this book at the International Longevity Center, one of our colleagues told a story about an aging man who maintained a high quality of life throughout his many years: At ninety-five, Frank Adams could have a been poster boy for morbidity compression. His story is worth retelling.

FRANK'S STORY. Along with his wife of more than sixty years, Frank lived in the farmhouse where he was born. He seemed amazingly active and alive despite his advanced age; the colleague who knew him was just a schoolboy then, delivering the local newspaper, but even now he remembers Mr. Adams having a good word for him every afternoon and, on collection day, an extra nickel tip (during the Kennedy administration, that meant something to an eleven-year-old). For the paperboy-turned-researcher many years later, the nostalgic recollection of a kindly old gentleman came to personify the idea of longevity.

Our colleague clearly enjoyed recalling the facts of a long life lived well. Yet perhaps he had another motive for repeating the story, a motive he himself did not altogether recognize. He told the story because deep down *he* wanted a long, healthy life like Mr. Adams. And in truth, examining the stories of the long-lived is one way to live longer yourself. In fact, within the simple recitation of Mr. Adams's life are a great many clues that can be of use to you in your quest for longevity and a high quality of life in the later years.

A series of follow-up questions about Mr. Adams further illuminate a simple boyhood recollection.

When asked what he usually saw Mr. Adams doing, our colleague shrugged, paused for recollection, then said, "I remember him working in the garden. Carrying in wood for the stove. Even snow shoveling."

Those few words confirm a truism of the longevity field: There is a strong correlation between an active life and a long one. So here was one of the keys to Mr. Adams's longevity: DAILY PHYSICAL ACTIVITY. Undoubtedly it contributed to his overall physical condition, too, as his young friend remembered him as slim and spry.

The mention of a garden prompted a question about what Mr. and Mrs. Adams cultivated. "There were vegetables, certainly, but I don't remember flowers," was the first recollection. After more thought, our friend recalled bright red tomatoes amid abundant foliage that seemed ready to climb over the fence. "And, *yes!*" he added quickly, "I remember a raspberry patch." When the boy had his tonsils out, Mrs. Adams had sent him a quart of frozen raspberries to soothe his sore throat.

We would need more evidence to be certain, of course, but even going on such small clues, we might surmise that the Adamses ate a HEALTHY DIET, one rich in vitamins, minerals, and fiber.

Mr. and Mrs. Adams were married; our informer was too young to understand the dynamics of their marriage (although, one hopes, theirs was a life of SHARED LOVE AND INTIMACY). But as a paperboy, he did know a bit about the Adams family: Another customer on his route was the Adamses' son and daughter-in-law who lived down the street, and the Adamses had an adult grandchild who lived in their town; our colleague later babysat for a great-grandchild. This evidence suggests that a NETWORK OF FAMILY SUPPORT was at hand.

The old man had once told him that he knew about delivering things, since for many years Mr. Adams had been a mail carrier. The broader implication of this fact is clear enough: Undoubtedly he had a broad-based SOCIAL NETWORK in his town, too.

Did he read the paper you delivered? With a laugh, our reporter said Mr. Adams usually buried his face in the paper even before his delivery boy could ride away, often with his pencil at the ready to do the crossword puzzle. He was obviously a man with an ACTIVE MIND.

Sometimes at delivery time Mr. Adams was to be found napping on the porch. A good thing, that: As we age, ADEQUATE SLEEP AND REST, at night and as naps, are essential to sustaining good health. His kindly manner with the boy? A fair interpretation of this would be that Mr. Adams exhibited an easy demeanor and, perhaps, a LOW LEVEL OF STRESS.

Frank Adams died quite a number of years ago, just shy of his one hundredth birthday. Yet looking back through the eyes of an eleven-year-old some forty years on, we were presented with a case study that personifies so much of what hundreds of geriatric specialists have observed, quantified, studied, and reported on in their clinical practices in the years since. Instinctively the not-quite-retired Mr. Adams ate well, maintained a healthy weight, and lived a physically active life. His small-town world offered him the rich rewards of love, family, and community; his intellect sought to understand the larger world and kept his mind active. He did not smoke, experienced little stress, and unabashedly took a nap when he needed one. In short, he lived a life with many pleasures, relatively few pains, and achieved an overall quality of life to which many of us aspire.

Today, we understand vastly more about the mechanism of aging than Mr. Adams's doctor did. We now see connections between the decline of the immune system and the incidence of cancer. New medical treatments and procedures today allow people who suffer heart attacks, strokes, and other potentially catastrophic health events to recover lost function. Most important of all, we have identified a range of risk factors that, if eliminated or reduced, can delay or even prevent the onset of disease. As a result, *compression of morbidity* has become an achievable goal for more than the lucky few. You will encounter many stories in the coming pages of people who, like Frank Adams, have made lifestyle decisions to enhance their longevity, to embrace the three-decade dividend.

navigating the news

The vast and growing literature on aging ranges from medical journals to lifestyle magazines for the general public. Television shows and countless books offer advice ranging from the wise to the witless. The most reliable sources are sound studies reported in medical journals and conducted by doctors, psychologists, epidemiologists, statisticians, and a range of other researchers. These draw thoughtful conclusions; in contrast, the least reliable findings tend to be the wide-ranging claims made on the basis of narrow or even nonexistent evidence.

A key task is to assess the validity of the latest claims.

Often there may be no intent to mislead, but lay journalists reporting on complex medical subjects do often distort (translation: *exaggerate*) the importance or the meaning of research findings. Engaging, punchy newspaper articles that make bold statements are more fun to read (and write) than those that qualify every little detail. People want to hear about the cure for cancer; the possibility that a new discovery might, way down the road, lead to good news makes a much less appealing story.

All of which puts the obligation on you to be a careful reader, listener, and watcher. But parsing the prose in order to smell the real science is not that hard. Here are three little guidelines that can help you be a better-informed reader— and a better advocate for your own health.

Get the whole story. By definition, a headline is a simplification. There is no room for qualifiers and, very often, the writer of the piece who carefully crafted it for scientific accuracy did not write the headline (an editor who never got past the second paragraph probably did).

Look at the numbers. A thorough report of a study should include at least a sampling of the statistics. See how many people participated in a study and over what duration; a finding based upon thousands of patients over a period of years is likely to be more definitive than a small, short-term study. The latter can be valid, too, of course, but is more likely to be argument for more research to confirm, disprove, or elaborate on the findings.

Go to the source. The Internet is an invaluable tool for collecting information. If you read about a new study in the paper or hear about it on the news, see if you can find the full text online. Or, at least, read what other journalists have reported. Learning a little jargon can make this material accessible: Mastering words like *risk* (danger), *incidence* (how frequently something occurs), *onset* (when a disease started), and other investigator vocabulary is not so hard.

Before you follow up with your physician demanding that a new treatment be prescribed for you, do your homework. That will enable you to have an intelligent discussion with the doctor and make you a better partner in your health care.

Embracing Life

Strictly speaking, longevity is measured in numbers: It is the arithmetical accumulation of days, weeks, months, and years that produces our chronological life. Yet aging—or, more accurately, its converse, staying young—is in no small measure a state of mind that defies measurement.

In the nineteenth century, Ralph Waldo Emerson observed, "We do not grow old. We grow young." The Sage of Concord obviously remained young in the best sense: Emerson was engaged and curious, alive to ideas and to the people and the world around him. The numbers mattered less to him than the intangibles.

Bernard Baruch—a man of Wall Street and Washington, who lived to ninety-four—expressed something of the same sentiment when he remarked, "Old age is always fifteen years older than I am."

I understand all too well that not everyone takes such a positive view. Not so long ago, aging was understood to involve a gradual withdrawal from society (psychologists called it *disengagement* or *interiority*). Such a separation no longer seems inevitable: How about businessman T. Boone

Pickens? At eighty-one the oilman reinvented himself as an advocate of alternative types of energy. Or Paul Volcker? At eighty-two, more than twenty years after retiring as chairman of the Federal Reserve, he was back in the saddle as chairman of President Barack Obama's Economic Recovery Advisory Board. Volcker and Pickens are not unique: Many individuals in their eighties or nineties shape the way millions of people think about our world.

Another figure in contemporary American culture has wise words to offer about the acceptance of aging. Two-time Academy Award–winning actress, writer, activist, and philanthropist Jane Fonda observes, "I'm aging and no one prepared me for what I would find. When I turned sixty, I realized I was entering my 'third act'—a time in my life to look back and put it all together and add it all up. I turned seventy in 2007, and I'm ready to dig much deeper into the aging process and understand what is going on in minds and bodies."

As a woman who seems to have defied the aging process for years, she has come to embrace aging, not to deny its reality. "We should accept what is happening as we age and not fear death or loss of youth." Aging, she thinks, is about not only acceptance but recognition. "Whatever has happened to us, we can't change, but we can change our attitudes and state of mind. All the centenarians I have met are at peace with their lives. It is a beautiful thing." Fonda is serious about reaching new understandings: She's at work on a book about her "third act."

No matter how positive our view of the aging process, it will be accompanied by growing fears. We worry about our bodies and our minds. We wonder about our ability to take care of ourselves in the coming years, about our mobility, mental flexibility, and what the aging process means for our independence. The fears are both appropriate and, in most cases, exaggerated. In the aging years, few of us get stronger, quicker, or cleverer (and those that do, for the most part, are recouping premature losses). But the aging years simply do not have to be a steep slide to mental and physical disability.

Longevity, in many ways, is a state of mind. Consider the results of a recent survey conducted by Yale University epidemiologist Becca Levy. Levy reported in 2002 that the perception of aging had a clear impact on longevity: Among the fifty-plus Ohio residents in her study, those who had positive perceptions of aging lived longer—*seven and a half years* longer. This bonus was greater than that associated with regular exercise and not smoking. The message is quite clear: If you think negatively about aging, then the aging years are a time of decline. If you resist, your chances of remaining healthier and happier as you age are measurably greater.

Another important study on aging was conducted by the MacArthur Foundation and summarized in a fine book called *Successful Aging* by John W. Rowe, M.D., and Robert L. Kahn, Ph.D. Rowe, Kahn, and company found that two strong predictors for high *physical* function in the eighth decade of life were higher *mental* function, the other the presence of *emotional support*. In short, an active mind and an engaged emotional life "help keep the aging body vital."

Think about it. It will do you good.

The Longevity Index

In an attempt to tailor your longevity prescription to your individual needs, we have assembled a simple tool we call the Longevity Index. It will help locate your personal predictors for longevity, the characteristics that medical, epidemiological, psychological, demographic, and other researchers have identified as reliable predictors of longevity. No such summary can be regarded as a precise instrument—none of the widely publicized biometric and psychometric assessments, despite claims to the contrary, truly is—but this is nonetheless an invaluable tool for helping put together a list of key changes that might lengthen your life and keep you healthy enough to enjoy living it.

Take the test and prepare to make some changes.

THE LONGEVITY INDEX

Read the following statements.

For those that are true, give yourself 3 points.
For those largely correct, add 2 points.
If one only partly applies, add 1 point.
If it is not all true for you, add 0 points.

1. I eat only modest amounts of foods high in saturated fats. I consume two to four daily servings of fruit; three to five servings of vegetables; and eat multiple portions of unprocessed grains, beans, or other fiber-rich foods daily.

2. I exercise at least five times per week. Three or more of my workouts involve continuous aerobic activity (e.g., walking, running, swimming); at least two involve resistance training that emphasizes weight-bearing exercise and range of motion.

3. My body mass index (BMI) is less than 25 (see *Body Mass Index*, page 141).

4. I sleep with a minimum of interruption seven or eight hours per night; I nap once a day for twenty to thirty minutes.

5. I am in a marriage/partnership with someone I trust and love and with whom I share physical intimacies.

6. I am in regular and agreeable contact with siblings, children, and extended family.

7. I maintain active friendships, some of them of many years duration; I care about these old friends.

8. I interact daily with a range of people, both in person and by phone or via e-mail. Three or more times a week I leave my home for social interactions with friends or family.

9. In the last year, I have made at least one new friend, a person with whom I communicate regularly.

10. I am neither depressed nor prone to prolonged bouts of anxiety. I do not obsessively relive unhappy moments in the past; I have a hopeful attitude for the future.

11. I continue to challenge myself to learn new things.

12. I keep up with the events in my immediate world and the world at large. I read magazines or newspapers; I listen to the news on the radio or television; I am aware of the goings-on in my immediate neighborhood and community.

13. I find simple joys in my life that lift my spirits. I laugh a good deal: at myself, at jokes, or with my friends.

14. I regularly do something that stretches my mental muscles: crosswords, sudoku or other puzzles, cards, chess, trivia, or other games; I read at least six books a year.

15. I do not harbor old grievances; I make adjustments to adapt to changing circumstances and advancing age; I accept life's losses and look to new challenges.

16. I have stress reduction strategies—such as yoga, tai chi, golf, gardening, meditation—that I employ to reduce anxiety or pressure.

17. I have come to recognize that experience, wisdom, perspective, and patience are all human qualities enhanced by age.

18. I consult my physician regularly for checkups, medication monitoring, appropriate periodic screening tests, and immunizations.

19. I take a daily multivitamin and mineral supplement, but do not take excessive amounts of individual vitamins. I also take one children's aspirin (81 mg) a day.

20. If medication has been prescribed for hypertension, high cholesterol, diabetes, or other chronic ailments, I take it as instructed.

21. I do self-exams on my breasts or testicles and am alert for changes in moles or birthmarks.

(continued on next page)

22. If I have experienced hearing or vision loss, I have acquired glasses or hearing aids that enable me to see and communicate.
23. I wear a seat belt and bicycle helmet and use sunblock as appropriate.
24. I do not smoke. *(If you do, deduct 5 points from your total.)*
25. I use alcohol only in moderation. As a woman, I consume no more than one drink (1½ ounces of alcohol) a day; or, as a man, I drink no more than 3 ounces of alcohol daily.

SCORING

Add your 1s, 2s, and 3s for each of the twenty-five questions.

TOTAL: 30 or below
Your health is in jeopardy. You must make constructive changes in your life-style to enhance longevity.

TOTAL: 31 to 50
Your instincts are good, but some judicious changes could pay significant dividends in terms of a longer, healthier life.

TOTAL: 51 to 60
Acceptable. But this is your life, so why not live it even better—and longer?

TOTAL: 61 or more
Impressive. But keep reading: Your life probably will be long, but there still may be some changes you can make to help enhance its quality.

five changes

The ball is in your court. Having answered the twenty-five lifestyle questions, which five answers do you need to change to increase your chances for longevity? You will learn more in the coming pages, but chances are you can already pencil in a few targets for yourself.

Make yourself a preliminary list, but consider identifying a mix of changes. One might be a dietary shift, another a reasonable resolution regarding physical activity. How about a regular game or task that will sharpen your thinking and a social goal and a volunteer task, too? It is never too soon to start adapting your life to take best advantage of the three-decade dividend.

1. _____

2. _____

3. _____

4. _____

5. _____

Once you know what to do, you can prepare for change.

LONGEVITY AWARENESS CHECK

Answer these four questions:

Q: *Are you a nonsmoker?*

Q: *Are you physically active?*

Q: *Is your alcohol consumption moderate (1 to 14 drinks per week)?*

Q: *Do you consume at least five servings daily of fruits and vegetables?*

If you answered no to all four questions, you are almost *four times* more likely to die sometime in the next decade.

That was the finding of a study, published in 2008, conducted by the Medical Research Council at Cambridge University (England). The study subjects—20,000 healthy men and women with no known cancers, heart disease, or circulatory problems—were between the ages of forty-five and seventy-nine. Over an eleven-year span, researchers found that those who lived the healthiest lifestyles were effectively *fourteen years younger* than those with four unhealthy behaviors.

Bottom line? No smoking, regular exercise, moderate alcohol consumption, and ample fruits and vegetables in the diet add up to a longer life. The Cambridge study offers a good baseline to longevity strategies.

My commitment in these pages is to provide you with prescriptive advice that will genuinely influence your health status and longevity. In 2009 I testified before the U.S. Senate Committee on Health, Education, Labor and Pensions, and my subject was the same, namely healthy aging. I would suggest that even before you consider the multiple strategies outlined in the nine chapters to follow that you consider the seven key features of aging as I laid them out for the senators. These uncomplicated guidelines are, in essence, the distillation of the findings of thousands of studies.

Follow these instructions, and you will likely live a longer and healthier life:

1. *Go for a walk.* If you can, do it every day for thirty minutes or more. Researchers find that a daily constitutional is characteristic among populations of centenarians. To put it another way: Physical fitness reduces your risk of dying young, so seek to find a workable mix of exercise that will help you improve your balance, flexibility, posture, and aerobic health.

2. *Watch your weight.* This means consuming a diet rich in fruits and vegetables (aim for 7 or even 9 servings per day), low in fat, with plenty of vitamin D, and one that keeps your weight within the normal range (see *Body Mass Index,* page 141).

3. *Reduce stress.* A healthy immune system, full cognitive function, and an overall sense of well-being depend upon managing the pressures in your life. Employ meditation, yoga, visualization, mini-vacations, appropriate sleep, and other strategies.

4. *Quit smoking.* If you are a smoker, your bargain with the nicotine fiend will cost you five, ten, or more years of life. So quit—no other single change presages such benefits.

5. *Avoid excessive alcohol consumption.* Men should consume fewer than two drinks a day (preferably one) and women no more than one. Such restrictions have been shown repeatedly to decrease many health risks.

6. *Build a strong social network.* A support system of friends can be invaluable not only in dealing with life's challenges but by enhancing daily life.

7. *Find a focus.* A sense of purpose—something to get up for in the morning—is part of the recipe for longevity. National Institutes of Health studies I contributed to in the 1950s and 1960 demonstrated even then that those individuals with a sense of purpose lived longer and better lives.

Finally, play the odds. Be sensible and wear your seat belt at all times when in an automobile and your helmet on a bicycle or motorcycle. Avoid excessive sun exposure. Use the medical system, too, getting regular checkups with your physician, who will recommend appropriate inoculations, screening tests (mammograms, colonoscopies, and others) to keep you healthy.

Read on. Learn more. The prescription works.

A word is just a word, of course, and no word can be truly good or bad. Words have no smell or other sensory reality beyond their sound and, if printed, the ink and paper with which they are represented. Yet words can be used as weapons to hurt or as shields to protect.

Words may not be alive, but they change and evolve, with meanings added as old ones fade. Words can be stigmatized, too, and one that has assumed a role in our world in recent years is *denial*. The word represents the refusal of people to recognize a perceived truth: People who deny their alcoholism, for example, are avoiding a painful reality; or denial can be a refusal to cope with responsibility or guilt.

Denial often poses a danger. It can be a form of lying or self-delusion that damages relationships. A denial of health symptoms can be life threatening: For the person suffering a heart attack, a denial of tightness in the chest may delay treatment and lead to unnecessary death. If we can agree that denial is a destructive and unhealthy behavior in most of its guises, then perhaps our health would be best served by acknowledging an important reality.

Namely, that we are aging.

Go ahead, say it: *I am aging.* Let's not deny that we are aging. Let's deal with it, accept it, and use it.

Aging has many qualities: It can bring wisdom, patience, and a reduced need to show off, to be seen, or to be heard. The pace of the aging years may be such that you find yourself thinking a little more deeply about things. There may be personal, professional, social, or even spiritual insights.

Might the relevant word here be *wisdom*?

The essence of wisdom is understanding. One of the ironies of life is that the people with the most time—the young—are always in the biggest hurry. The wise elder appreciates that speed in most of its guises is overrated.

Time adds a dimension to our understanding of ourselves and the world around us. It amounts to a sort of critical distance that enables us to see possibilities: deeper layers; the capacity to change; that beyond the obvious are less tangible yet potentially more meaningful aspects. For some it is spiritual; for others it is emotional; for still others it is about connections.

Quantifying the wisdom we gain as we age has proved elusive, but investigators have tried and, to some degree, succeeded. A notable attempt has been the Berlin Aging Study. For more than twenty years, the researchers have been looking at positive aspects of human aging. In particular, their hope has been to find that wisdom comes with age. In fact, the ongoing research suggests that age alone does not bring wisdom, but that the wise person recognizes value and significance; excellence and the common good are goals.

We can use our wisdom to identify what we desire in our lives: To improve ourselves, our lives, our health, our relationships, enhance our longevity, and to amend our lifestyle; all of these are central to this book, to what we call the Longevity Prescription. Extending your healthy years is about using proven, practical strategies to live well during what physicians call the "post-meridian phase" of life. These approaches have been developed by internationally recognized gerontologists, epidemiologists, physiologists, psychiatrists, and sociologists, along with a range of other researchers, physicians, and public health professionals. The following pages contain authoritative, accessible, and practical advice, which adds up to a prescription for maximum physical, intellectual, and emotional health during the aging years, a means of cashing in on the three-decade dividend.

This programmatic approach—that is, the *prescription* promised in this book's title—is not a magic pill or a daily dose of the elixir from the fountain of youth (if only continued good health were so simple). Rather, *The Longevity Prescription* seeks to engage you in a process by which your understanding of longevity science informs the way you live your life. Some of the best clinicians, scientists, physicians, and researchers in the world are focusing their energies on understanding aging, but your commitment to living long and well is required to employ a selection of the strategies described in these pages.

The choices are many. Some will help maximize your memory and others build up your biceps, but not every strategy suits every individual. In the chapters that follow, you will learn about stress, social and intimate involvements, sleep, and other matters that have a powerful and direct impact on the aging process. You will need to make changes, to discipline yourself to reach out and embrace new activities.

A plan will emerge, a prescription for a longer, healthier life.

PRESCRIPTION I

MAINTAIN MENTAL VITALITY

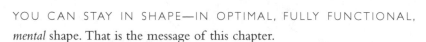

YOU CAN STAY IN SHAPE—IN OPTIMAL, FULLY FUNCTIONAL, *mental* shape. That is the message of this chapter.

In talking to people every day about longevity, I find their greatest fear is of losing their minds. This is the era of Alzheimer's disease, and according to current polling data, the potential for an Alzheimer's diagnosis intimidates us the way that heart disease once did. Even though there is no preventative for Alzheimer's (I wish there was), new scientific findings demonstrate that you can take steps to resist what we physicians like to call cognitive decline.

The term *cognition* is used to describe what your brain does as it reasons, remembers, and processes perceptions. Your *cognitive capacity* is your ability with language, learning, and memory. Cognition includes mental functions that enable you to pay attention, plan your day, make good judgments, and execute skilled motor behaviors. Cognitive function affects a person's ability to interact and enjoy life, and research shows that, as individuals, we can influence mental health status as we age.

To avoid cognitive decline, you must work to keep your mental functions alive and well. From personal experience, we all know the muscles and bones and other organs lose some of their youthfulness with age. In the same way, cognitive function declines somewhat in the aging years, as the rate at which the brain receives and processes information slows. This can also lead to memory loss.

A number of studies have demonstrated that this decline is neither inevitable nor as severe as many people think. About 80 percent of older people report memory loss—but testing has found that such subjective reports are overstated. It appears that our *fear* of a fading memory exaggerates real but minor memory loss. While mental functions often seem to slow with age, the cognitive changes associated with normal aging generally are mild and will not impair the ability to function on a day-to-day basis.

Know this, too: Cognitive impairments of aging are potentially avoidable using the strategies that follow. Making it a priority to employ them can enhance your cognitive vitality.

Cognitive Vitality

Researchers in longevity science are developing a new conceptual approach to maintaining cognitive vitality. An example of the new understandings that underlie this work was published in 2006 in the *Journal of the American Medical Association*. The investigators reported on a study that examined the impact of training older adults in memory, reasoning, and mental processing. The participants were over age sixty-five, living independently, and functioning well in their day-to-day lives.

The training was not difficult. In sixty- to seventy-five-minute sessions, three groups were given memory strategies for organizing, visualizing, or associating verbal material such as word lists; reasoning training, such as finding patterns in letter or word series; and speed-of-processing training (one drill involved identifying an object on a computer screen at increasingly brief exposures). For purposes of comparison, some participants in this blind trial were given no training.

The results were impressive—and encouraging. Those who received the ten sessions of training saw their cognitive abilities improve. The benefit was measurable, immediate, and long-lasting, as the trial found that gains made in reasoning, memory, and speed of mental processing were still very much in evidence five years later.

Even better, other assessments conducted by the researchers determined that the cognitive training had practical value, too, in what psychologists call the "instrumental activities of daily living." In comparison to the control group, the participants in the study who had received cognitive training retained more independence and were less likely to require hospital, outpatient, home health, and home nursing services.

The message is clear: You can take responsibility for keeping your brain in optimal condition.

❋

NOLA OCHS DID. She was a full-time student at Fort Hays State University in Kansas during the academic year 2006–2007. She was older than her classmates, as her studies had been interrupted by family affairs and the obligations of running the family wheat farm after her husband died. But for her senior year at Hays State, she decided to devote herself full-time to her studies. She resided in an on-campus apartment and researched her papers online like other college students in today's Internet-connected world.

What is remarkable is that Ms. Ochs, who received her degree in history on May 12, 2007, did so at age *ninety-five*, becoming the oldest recorded college graduate.

The chair of FHSU's history department admitted to initial doubts as to whether Ochs could keep up with the other students. Just two weeks into the semester, he set aside his concerns. "To have Nola in a class adds a dynamic that can't be topped," he said. She shared with the class her recollections of the Depression-era Dust Bowl, bringing a human side to bloodless textbook paragraphs about the past.

Like many of her classmates (among them was Alexandra Ochs, one of her thirteen grandchildren), Nola Ochs had her eye on the horizon. "I plan to seek employment on a cruise ship," she told Jay Leno with a twinkle, "going around the world as a storyteller."

I recommend you do as Nola did and make a plan to challenge your brain.

Making Changes

In the absence of severe brain disease, humans do not stop developing, whatever our age. If you can read and absorb the words on this page, you can adjust, improve, and amend the way you live to enhance your chances of enjoying the three-decade dividend.

Researchers are publishing new findings all the time. Investigators in 2009 reported on how the brains of both humans and laboratory rodents experience *neurogenesis* throughout life. In layman's terms, neurogenesis is the process by which your brain continues to regenerate nerve cells, including neurons and other so-called neural lineages. The process is not as rapid in the mature central nervous system as it is in a child's, but the adult human brain is constantly adapting and even reprogramming itself.

One aspect of ongoing research concerns *neuroplasticity*, the ability of the brain throughout life to reorganize neural pathways based on new experiences. New clinical studies are exploring how subjective experience—what you did yesterday, for example—affects your mental processes today. The research in this area is varied and complex; some of it utilizes controversial stem cells (both adult and newborn); and the work is happening at sites as far-flung as Johns Hopkins University in Baltimore, and Dharamsala, India. But revolutionary findings demonstrate that at the molecular level, social and intellectual experiences have an impact on the function of your brain.

At the International Longevity Center, we initiate and monitor new research, and we see much that is of practical value to you. Many of the newest findings suggest you can transition from old habits to new, healthier ones. Studies in human populations have found repeatedly that there are three key predictors of healthy mental function in the later years: a can-do attitude, a support system of family and friends, and physical activity. Each of these is under your control. If you make a set of strategic changes—we'll talk about three sets of changes in coming pages—you can build your confidence. You can enlist family and friends to help (in *Prescription II: Nurture Your Relationships*, page 57, we will offer guidance as to how to go about that). When it comes to exercise, you will find practical steps to take in *Prescription VI: Live the Active Life* (see page 138).

Did you know that men and women who have experienced a decline in cognitive ability can, with training, regain as much as two decades of memory? Healthy lifestyle modifications, even the small ones, will benefit you, as long as they are performed on a regular basis. It is never too late to stimulate those brain cells.

Strategy One: Cognitive Calisthenics

The task is to exercise the brain's remarkable flexibility. The more you employ your knowledge base, language skills, planning, judgment, attention, concentration, and skilled motor behaviors, the better conditioned your brain will be. "Lifetime learning" may have become a cliché, but ongoing mental challenges can be life-enhancing and even life-giving. As with physical fitness, mental vitality comes with conditioning. It is time for a revitalization.

THE ASSIGNMENT. My prescription is as follows:

1. Find an activity that challenges your brain.
2. Invest a minimum of twenty minutes a day, at least five days a week, in that activity.

3. Monitor your progress weekly to be sure you follow through and to reinforce your success and enjoyment.
4. Over time, move to harder puzzles, more difficult reading materials, or more challenging tasks.

THE ACTIVITIES. The following are suggested activities; the list is extensive but by no means comprehensive.

- *Turn off the television.* For one hour each evening, read a newspaper, magazine, or a book instead of putting your mind in neutral as you watch TV.
- *Bookmark your favorite website.* Maybe it's the op-ed page of *The New York Times* or a favorite blogger. Identify a daily stimulus that gets the mental gears turning. Read, absorb, think, and discuss.
- *Learn a word a day.* Improve your vocabulary. Pick a word out of the paper or the dictionary every day, put it on an index card, and drill yourself.
- *Revisit a book.* Reread a favorite. Find one by an author you know but have not read yet. Better yet, take a chance and expand your universe.
- *Buy an e-book.* If you're a voracious reader tired of carrying heavy books around, buy an electronic reading device. The Amazon Kindle and Sony Reader are the best known. About the thickness of a magazine and weighing less than pound, they have screens roughly the size of a rack-size paperback. Capable of holding hundreds or even thousand of books, these devices start at about $200.
- *Learn to play the guitar.* Or take up the piano, clarinet, cello, or some other instrument. Take lessons, establish a daily practice schedule, and stay with it. Join a choir or take singing lessons.
- *Memorize a poem.* Start with a short one that pleases you. If it is fun, move on to a longer poem, maybe one that tells a story.

- *Subscribe to a newspaper or magazine.* Online or by snail mail, get in the habit of reading a periodical that covers subjects that interest you.
- *Learn a new language.* Start with tapes, or take a class. Use it as an incentive to plan a trip. It will be challenging but worth it.
- *Become computer literate.* If you have not already, learn how to surf the net or play a brain-challenging game (see *Products to Train Your Brain*, page 31).
- *Play puzzles.* Most daily newspapers have crossword puzzles, and many have acrostics, sudoku, KenKen, or other games.
- *Pursue a passion.* Is there something you have always dreamed of trying, like oil painting, poetry writing, or bird-watching? Get a book out the library, find a mentor, search the Web, take a class, check the Yellow Pages. Find a way to scratch that old itch.

A WORD TO THE WISE. Hard mental work produces benefits. Studies of intellectual function and memory decline among the aging have shown that when older persons are presented with difficult problems, they score much better than when they are tested with trivial ones. Have fun and enjoy what you do—but keep in mind that challenges that truly improve your mind may deliver the most benefit.

deciding to decide

You are of sound mind, healthy body, and looking to assure that remains the case. Ironically, that also means you should also be weighing your options for future life changes.

Anticipation is wonderful skill: No one can see the future, of course, but planning, flexibility, and a willingness to consider hard choices can have a large impact on your quality of life in the future. Lots of people decide not to decide (researchers call this *ambiguity aversion*), but a refusal to consider the future may mean narrowed options or, worse, no choice at all. If you're like most people, time seems to accelerate as we get older, which makes thinking about your future all the more important. It will be upon you before you know it.

Think about choices. Eventually you will have to make certain major decisions—some of the likely ones concern retirement, altering your living circumstances, and end-of-life care—and I think you will find that a decision is easier when you already have a little perspective on the subject. The way to get that is by accumulating a little knowledge—from friends, professional advisors, magazines, books, the Internet, wherever—and by having some open-minded discussion with your spouse or partner, family members, and other counselors. The need to make a change may seem less shocking if you've already established a framework for considering it by talking and thinking about options over a period of years.

Talk about retirement. Retirement is a perfect case in point. It is a decision—*to retire or not to retire*—that almost everyone faces at some time. If you work at a salaried job, your decision may be partly decided for you by your benefits (Do they improve with longer tenure? Are there thresholds such as age sixty-two or sixty-five where the incentive to retire increases?). Generous or not, the retirement plan you have will likely set certain parameters for your decision.

Whether or not you can expect a pension, shape scenarios in your mind: What would your life be like if you retired tomorrow? Or ten years from now? Be realistic about income and expenses; compare that future to the present. If the picture looks bleak, that's not an argument for ending the discussion; on the contrary, you need to find ways to brighten the picture. Reach out: There are family, friends, and professional counselors who can help you make a plan, to make changes that can help assure a more comfortable future. But you need to have the conversations.

Look into new locations. Another decision set has to do with where you live. Relocating to another part of the country is one variable; another sort is the move to a different kind of living accommodation. During the aging years, some people decide to downscale in size, or to move from a single-family house to an apartment or condominium where maintenance responsibilities fall to someone else. Further down the road, a retirement community, an assisted-living facility, or other kinds of care facilities may be appropriate.

Your odds for longevity increase with your ability to assess your needs, wishes, and overall health and to align them with your circumstances. Be optimistic but not unrealistic. Think about stages: Knowing what you do today about your health, family, and working life, where might you reasonably expect to be at, say, ages sixty-five, seventy, seventy-five, or eighty? Keep in mind you are looking at a moving target, one that can have stops in more than one safe harbor along the way.

Don't expect time to solve your problems: Planning your journey or, at the very least, thinking and talking about it, will be valuable to you.

The Vital Pursuit of Happiness

His first seventy years were remarkable enough. A child of Depression-era Tennessee and the first in his town to go to college, John Templeton finished first in his class at Yale. He was awarded a Rhodes Scholarship, studied at Oxford's Balliol College, then embarked on a wildly successful career as a global investor and founder of Templeton Mutual Funds.

At age seventy, he established the Templeton Prize for Progress in Religion; at seventy-five he established the Templeton Foundation; and a month before his eightieth birthday, he sold his mutual fund empire (assets: $22 billion) in order to devote his time to his philanthropies. He lived another fifteen years, dying in 2008 at age ninety-five.

Though he was a lifelong Presbyterian, he was a seeker, a man curious about other faiths. He believed in what he called spiritual progress. He once asked an interviewer, "Why shouldn't I go to Hindu services? Why shouldn't I go to Muslim services? If you are not egotistical, you will welcome the opportunity to learn more."

The self-made billionaire devoted his aging years to the pursuit not of

PRODUCTS TO TRAIN YOUR BRAIN

Nature is not alone in abhorring a vacuum: So do entrepreneurs. In the new world of neuroplasticity, lots of writers, software engineers, publishers, gamers, and others are producing products. The books, games, "neurosoftware," and other products promise "brain training" that will help you stimulate your prefrontal cortex, improve your mental acuity, and generally keep your brain agile. Some of these claims are undoubtedly overstated, but at the very least there are fun and stimulating workouts for your brain to be found in some of the products on the market.

Books. Among the books are Sharon Begley's *Train Your Mind, Change Your Brain: How a New Science Reveals Our Extraordinary Potential to Transform Ourselves*, which looks at the Dalai Lama, Buddhists, and researchers to understand the ways in which in they have been able to alter brain function. The title of another book describes its contents: *The Brain That Changes Itself: Stories of Personal Triumph from the Frontiers of Brain Science* by Norman Doidge, a Canadian psychiatrist. Perennial how-to favorites include *Keep Your Brain Alive: 83 Neurobic Exercises* by Lawrence Katz and Manning Rubin, and *Brain Builders! A Lifelong Guide to Sharper Thinking, Better Memory, and an Age-Proof Mind* by Richard Leviton.

Neurosoftware. New products continue to arrive on the market; among those available are *Posit Science's Brain Fitness Program*, consisting of computer-based exercises to improve memory and other mental functions; *MindFit* ("a personal trainer for your brain"); and the Nintendo-based game *Brain Age: Train Your Brain in Minutes a Day*, which is described as a "treadmill for the mind" (actually a series of mini-games designed for use with Nintendo's hand-held DS system; *Brain Challenge* and *Brain Voyage* are others).

The Internet. Wander the Web, where sites such as BrainBuilder.com, SharpBrains.com, and Luminosity.com offer information, products, and, in some cases, free trials. Try a search using *brain training, memory games,* and other key words. Keep in mind that the discipline of seeking information, on the Web and otherwise, is in itself an intellectual exercise that can help sharpen memory, reasoning, and mental processing skills.

money but of happiness in a context that was both spiritual and scientific. His foundation awards grants to scientists concerned with religious claims about the cosmos or human destiny; the focus is on science, but in the realm of religious rituals, prayer, charity, and faith.

Despite a chorus of critics, Templeton saw no paradox in mixing theology and science; that was what intrigued him. The Templeton Prize has gone to figures as varied as Mother Teresa, Aleksandr Solzhenitsyn, Billy Graham; to Hindu, Buddhist, and Hebrew scholars; and to mathematicians, theologians, cosmologists, and scientists concerned with the environment, physics, genetics, and other fields.

Science can no more explain religion than faith can make the cosmos intellectually comprehensible. But as Sir John (Queen Elizabeth awarded him a knighthood in 1987) believed, asking big questions in an open-minded and humble way is important. Money cannot buy longevity, but Sir John's embracing view of life probably helped him sustain a long, creative, and stimulating life. His example, which can be useful to all of us, is summed up in the motto of his foundation: "How little we know, how eager to learn."

Memory

I have heard all manner of stories, including the one about the woman who lost her cell phone, only to find it later in her freezer. And the anecdote about the fellow who drove to work one day then took the bus home— only to wonder where his car was. How about the lady who showed up at the doctor's office and discovered that she was supposed to be at the dentist?

When we hear them second or third hand, these little moments can be amusing. Then one day you cannot seem to attach a name to a familiar face or remember a term you called up from your mental dictionary just last week. Then your keys go missing.

First, there is no reason for panic. Almost everyone in the aging years experiences a decline in memory.

Second, resolve to get your memory in shape. But before we look at more strategies for mnemonic stimulation, let's look at how the memory works.

HOW WE REMEMBER. According to new scientific insights into the workings of the brain, our recollections seem to be organized by the way we collect and use them.

The primary or working memory contains the information needed for the tasks at hand. An example would be reading this chapter, even this paragraph. As you read, you take in the content and absorb just enough into your *working memory* to understand what you have read before you move on.

Your *secondary memory* organizes and stores information in order for you to be able to access it over a long period of time. Thus, if you go to the trouble to memorize the elements of this discussion and can explain them to someone next month or next year, the information in these paragraphs has become secondary memory.

Secondary memory, in turn, is divisible into *explicit* and *implicit* memory. Conscious recollections are explicit. Explicit memories can be subdivided still further: the autobiographical pieces in your explicit memory are called *episodic memory*, while *semantic memories* concern historical, academic, and generalized knowledge.

If this seems confusing, the message is not: Your working memory is likely to be little affected by aging. We carry on our daily routines with little disruption as we age, using the habits and procedures stowed in our implicit memories.

UNDERSTANDING MEMORY DECLINE. During the aging years, the explicit secondary memory is more likely to show signs of fading. This is reflected in what people now call "noun loss," in which we cannot remember the name of the actress who starred in the movie we saw last week or the author of a recently reviewed book. Studies have shown a similar decline in what psychologists call "delayed recall" as the decades pass. After reading two lengthy paragraphs, older people recalled less of what they read than younger people did.

Memory is not a single skill or ability, any more than intelligence is, and we depend upon memory for almost everything we do. Perhaps that is why no other symptom of aging intimidates people as much as memory loss. When the small type in the newspaper blurs, we buy glasses. When our cholesterol count elevates, we take a pill. We adjust our physical activities, too, to align with modest declines in flexibility, strength, stamina, and recovery time. But forgetfulness can be harder to take in stride.

THE BEAUTY OF FLEXIBILITY. The brain is highly flexible. The central nervous system is constantly processing a range of stimuli; its dynamic ability to adapt is just beginning to be understood by scientists. It appears that there is no one pathway for processing thought, but the circuitry in your brain is interconnected in multiple ways, resulting in what neurologists call *neural redundancy*. These are backup systems: When one goes does down, another is at hand to help carry the load.

This network is enhanced by mental activity. More than one study has found a relationship between higher educational levels and a reduced risk of age-related cognitive decline. Momentum is gathering behind the notion that the use-it-or-lose-it rule applies to the brain just as it does to the musculoskeletal system.

I like the story of James Smithson because it demonstrates what I'm talking about. Smithson hung up his professorial robes at age fifty-eight. While he still enjoyed the students after more than thirty years of teaching college biology, his patience with his faculty and administrative colleagues had grown thin. The department seemed less and less concerned with merit and ever more focused upon interoffice politics. So he took early retirement, planning to revise his textbooks, concentrate on collecting nineteenth-century Staffordshire pottery, and enjoy his greenhouse labors.

Within days of his sixtieth birthday, James felt a shiver of cold fear run through him. He was explaining to a guest how the begonias—his favorite plant family—are easily hybridized into new and unique plants called . . . well, called what? "I just couldn't bring the word up," he remembers. "I knew the term as well as my own name. I'd used it the day before but the word—it was 'cultivars,' of course—just seemed to have fallen out of my head."

Along with the blurring vision of middle age (the term for that is *presbyopia*), memory loss is a normal part of aging. But Professor Smithson resolved that he was not going to lose a lifetime's worth of accumulated learning. He made a game of memorizing ten words a day. He quizzed himself weekly. A math department friend recommended a British algebra text filled almost exclusively with word problems. He developed these and other strategies to keep his mind in shape.

It worked for him and today, ten years into his retirement, his mind is as active as ever.

LONGEVITY AWARENESS CHECK

Ask yourself these questions:

Q When people invite you to lunch, parties, or other events, how often do you politely decline?

Q When was the last time you looked up a word in the dictionary?

Q How long has it been since you went to a ball game, movie, or public performance?

Q When was the last time you made a new friend?

Having answered these questions honestly, consider one more:

Q Are you living life fully?

The vital life involves thinking and interacting as often and as vigorously as possible.

The Aging Brain

If you occasionally have difficulty recalling names or if minor recent events seem to have a way of slipping from your memory, then you are a member of a very large club. A closer look at the neurology of aging reveals ways in which the brain changes over time.

Cognition relies upon a network of billions of brain cells. Some links in that network break down as we age, and we need additional time to process and react to information. Often we are blithely unaware of these little changes because most daily activities do not test the limits of our ability to process information. However, the bottleneck of slowed processing can cause other shortcomings in cognitive function, such as memory lapses, in particular when we attempt to access multiple memories simultaneously in completing tasks.

There are literally thousands of day-to-day causes of forgetfulness. It is a simple fact, for example, that you are more likely to forget things when you are sick, stressed, or distracted. We may know instinctively that a poor night's sleep noticeably dulls most mental functions, but there is new research, published in the *Journal of Neuroscience*, that demonstrates sleep accelerates working memory performance.

Sometimes the causes of memory loss are more insidious. Uncontrolled inflammation is one possible explanation. Stress is another. A change in hormonal levels can be a factor, such as occurs with the cessation of estrogen production at menopause. In some people, depression is the cause, as is head trauma (just ask the quarterback who, his bell rung on second down, cannot remember the play call for third-and-long). Other causes may include excessive alcohol consumption, recreational drug use or prescription drug interactions, mini-strokes (multi-infarct), brain cancer, or Alzheimer's disease.

For most people, the elusive memories will be accessed in a matter of time; yesterday's mild forgetfulness is nothing to worry about, as it does not involve other cognitive functions and isn't likely to be progressive.

AGE-ASSOCIATED MEMORY IMPAIRMENT. Neurologists use the clinical acronym AAMI to describe the initial stage of more significant cognitive or mental decline. AAMI involves a generalized decline in the ability to perform tasks related to concentration and organization, as well as memory. AAMI tends to progress very slowly and is attributed to the normal aging process.

MILD COGNITIVE IMPAIRMENT (MCI). MCI is characterized by more serious memory deficits. It is regarded as a transition stage; while many people with MCI remain stable, others eventually develop Alzheimer's disease. Once called *benign senescent forgetfulness*, this stage is now understood in a more sinister light. Personality changes usually accompany the forgetfulness described by MCI, and studies done on cerebrospinal fluids obtained through spinal taps have found lower levels of substances associated with acetylcholine, dopamine, and serotonin, the brain transmitters that enable nerve-to-nerve communication. Imaging techniques such as positron emission tomography (PET) and magnetic resonance imaging (MRI) have identified tissue deterioration in the brain matter of subjects with mild cognitive impairment.

The dementia that may follow is not a normal part of aging. While most people develop some degree of cognitive decline after age seventy, many do not experience a steep decline and a great many very old people, including centenarians, maintain high cognitive function.

If you or someone you know experiences sudden and severe memory loss, especially if it is accompanied by other neurological problems, discuss the symptoms with a physician. Potential causes include many treatable medical conditions, including depression, vitamin deficiencies, hormonal imbalances, tumors, brain trauma, and AIDS. Medications associated with forgetfulness and confusion include the anti-inflammatory prednisone; sedatives such as triazolam, diazepam, and alprazolam; excessive doses of insulin (which cause hypoglycemia); some heartburn drugs, including cimetidine, famotidine, and ranitidine; and a number of medications used to treat cancer, heart disease, hypertension, Parkinson's disease, pain, and even the common cold. Alcohol is the single most common cause of confusion but, as with the medications, if you stop taking it, the loss of memory and intellectual function is likely to be reversed.

ALZHEIMER'S DISEASE. This ailment has became the chief fear of many aging people, not least because of its prevalence: Roughly one in twenty Americans over sixty-five is affected, and the number rises to more like one in three after age eighty.

A German physician named Dr. Alois Alzheimer first described the illness that bears his name. A female patient at the clinic where he worked in Frankfurt exhibited a loss of short-term memory at age fifty-one, and developed psychiatric symptoms, too, including disorientation and hallucinations. Dr. Alzheimer recorded her behavior prior to her premature death at age fifty-five, then examined her brain in a postmortem autopsy. He found tissues just as confused as she had been (he called the twisted fragments of protein he found in her nerve cells *neurofibrillary tangles*).

Much has been learned since her death 1907. We now understand that the regions most affected are deep in the brain. These cortical and subcortical areas, which include the hippocampus, are charged with regulating memory, attention, and other high thought processes. In patients with Alzheimer's disease, nerve-to-nerve communication, which occurs at connections called synapses, begins to fail. Several causes have been identified, including a shortfall of acetylcholine and other neurotransmitters, which are necessary for the activation of nerve receptors. Researchers have also observed that certain proteins are found in the unusually high densities of plaques, the fatty deposits of cholesterol and calcium associated with atherosclerosis, also characteristic of Alzheimer's patients. Inflammation in the brain has been implicated, too, yet the precise mechanism of the disease still remains unclear.

Some people are more likely than others to become Alzheimer's patients. Epidemiological evidence suggests that people most at risk are those with Down syndrome, a family history of dementia, previous head trauma, and possibly hypertension and a history of heart attack. The single biggest factor, however, is age: Growing old does not automatically put you on the road to Alzheimer's, but a disproportionate number of Alzheimer's sufferers are in their advancing years.

Diagnosis. The onset of Alzheimer's is characterized by a constellation of changes in behavior and function. Forgetting a name or a date probably isn't an indicator, though memory loss that disrupts daily life, such as regularly losing track of dates or events and asking for the same information repeatedly, may be. Also characteristic is difficulty in performing familiar tasks, such as executing a recipe, balancing a checkbook, participating in games, or following the route to a well-known destination. Difficulty in judging distance or identifying colors and losing the conversational thread are also typical, as is bad judgment in dealing with money and strangers. Social withdrawal, uncharacteristic mood changes, and an overall alteration of personality are also symptomatic of Alzheimer's disease.

Treatment. For the person diagnosed with Alzheimer's disease, a range of drug therapies may be useful. Since the loss of neurotransmitters, in particular acetylcholine, has been implicated in Alzheimer's disease, drugs such as rivastigmine and donepezil that inhibit the chemicals that destroy acetylcholine have been found to slow memory decline for a year or more. Other chemotherapeutic approaches such as memantine may work to enhance cognition.

Prevention. In the absence of a clearer understanding of Alzheimer's disease, the best strategy is to reduce the known treatable factors in the occurrence of the disorder, which include high blood pressure, diabetes, smoking, cardiovascular disease, and sleep apnea. In one study recently presented at an American Academy of Neurology conference, people at risk of Alzheimer's who consumed more than two drinks a day were found to have developed the disease almost five years earlier than those who drank less. The onset of Alzheimer's was more than two years earlier among heavy smokers (according to one study, the risk of Alzheimer's for smokers over sixty-five is 79 *percent greater* than nonsmokers). Thus, limiting alcohol consumption and quitting smoking may decrease your odds of contracting Alzheimer's disease.

There are promising avenues of research, including a British investigation of iron-binding drugs (iron has been found to accumulate in the brains of Alzheimer's patients) and ongoing explorations of so-called Alzheimer's genes. However, living a healthy lifestyle is the best we can do at present to decrease our odds of getting Alzheimer's. Get adequate sleep (the memory-and-rest connection is clear; see *Prescription III: Seek Essential Sleep,* page 83). Find time for plenty of exercise both mental and physical (see *Prescription I: Maintain Mental Vitality,* page 22, and *Prescription VI: Live the Active Life,* page 138). Since stress may also play a role, avoid making life a pressure cooker (see *Prescription IV: Set Stress Aside,* page 103). In short, following the Longevity Prescription is the best route to reducing your risk of Alzheimer's disease.

Strategy Two: Reconfigure Your Brain

The task is to think of your brain as a computer that you wish to update. The addition of some new hardware, perhaps an add-on or two, and you will be up to speed. If you can increase your interactions by engaging the human energy around you in new ways, you *can* revitalize your brain.

THE ASSIGNMENT. My recommendation is this:

1. Select an activity from the list that follows.
2. Devote at least one hour on each of two days of the week to pursing it; or
3. Identify a one-time task that is to be accomplished in a fixed period, such as thirty to ninety days. Then choose another one upon completing the first.

THE ACTIVITIES. Here are some choices:

- *Join a reading group.* You will get a book to read for each meeting and people with whom to talk about it.
- *Take a trip.* There is nothing like a change of scenery to make you think, to pique your curiosity, to open new avenues you did not know were there.
- *Make the journey an intellectual joy.* Before you go, find a book that relates to your destination: If it is to be Paris, there is Adam Gopnik's *Paris to the Moon*; for New York, Jack Finney's *Time and Again*. When in Florida, try a novel by Carl Hiaasen. How about Jane Austen's England?
- *Make entertaining a target.* Schedule dinner, lunch, or coffee hour regularly with friends.
- *Employ e-mail.* If you already have an e-mail account, check it regularly. Send news and notes to friends, new and old. If you're not an e-mailer yet, keep in mind that anybody can do it. Basic computer literacy comes surprisingly easily with new, not-so-expensive laptop computers.
- *Volunteer.* Hospitals, schools, retirement homes, and countless organizations are always looking for help. Whether your taste runs to tutoring, technology, the environment, politics, history, or the arts, there is probably a nearby organization that will welcome your time and energy.
- *Join a club.* Most groups are often seeking new members—if you like gardening, fishing, hiking, sewing, or dancing, there is probably a club out there for you. If there is no club that serves your particular interest, start one.
- *Write a family history.* Start with a family tree, then tell a story about each branch (see also *The Life Review*, page 43).

- *Collect something.* Maybe it is an old hobby from childhood; if you ever collected anything, it is probably easier now with the Internet. Find something that interests you—pottery, matchboxes, books, some sort of art, model cars, perfume bottles, whatever—and learn about it. Then go on a search that involves meeting and interacting with other collectors and dealers.
- *Relive your youth.* Revisit a passion from the past: woodworking, film noir, scouting, model trains, dog shows, quilting, Sunday school, playing sports—the list is as long and as varied as your life.
- *Plan and plant a vegetable garden.* The thinking, the exercise, the pursuit of seedlings, the gifting of the excess, the enjoyment of your produce—all will be health-giving.
- *Take up photography.* Thanks to digital technology, photographic images are easier than ever to make and manipulate as well as share with friends and family. Take a photography course or explore some of the technological possibilities. Or go retro and shoot real film; it remains a wonderful mode of artistic and personal expression.
- *Don't be afraid to play.* Children engage in play: It can be fun, silly, easy, and frivolous, as formless as a bout of tickling; or it can be structured (as in a game, with rules and expectations). Psychologists, anthropologists, sociologists, and even animal behaviorists have all examined play, observing its role in human development, relationships, society, technology, art, and the animal kingdom. Play also has a place—a very important place—in healthy aging.
- *Open your mind.* If you don't like something about your life, sit down and reframe your thinking; make a plan to change it. If life becomes a superhighway with no exits, you will miss a great deal of the landscape. Consider taking a different exit than usual. And consult *Prescription II: Nurture Your Relationships* (page 57) and *Prescription V: Connect with Your Community* (page 120).

A WORD OF ADVICE. The above suggestions are not your only choices: There are others out there that will suit you and engage your mind and spirit. Keep in mind that there is evidence that among people in their sixties and seventies their judgment, accuracy, and general knowledge may in fact increase if exercised; your assignment is to find a means or, better yet, two or three new ways to accomplish exactly that.

the more you know

Forgetfulness may have hidden virtues. In 2008, Shelley H. Carson, a psychologist conducting research at Harvard, explained the theory that in many older people, forgetfulness may actually be "distractibility."

The older we are, the more we have absorbed. The wider focus of attention that comes with having taken in more data can make it more difficult to pluck from the brain a particular fact like a name or a number; to put it another way, the more you know, the more cluttered your brain can become. At the same time, however, older people may be able to process a wider range of related data, which can make them better problem solvers. In various studies, young people have been found to be more likely to filter out distracting information; in comparison, older people are better at applying seemingly irrelevant things in original ways.

Is this wisdom? Some psychologists think so.

The Life Review

For more than fifty years, I have been exploring ways in which memories can be used as a health strategy. I have long believed that, in the later years, one of the normal tasks of a healthy person is to review life's events. An examination of such recollections may open the door to past conflicts, and a fresh look at such moments offers the opportunity to resolve them. We can integrate a mix of experiences and, in some cases, attain a new serenity.

The construction—and the reconstruction—of each life can become an act of celebration. As our life story nears completion, each of us has the opportunity to try to come to terms with its moral, personal, and emotional dimensions. The desire to look backward with an eye to reaching new understandings is hardly new, but when I helped initiate the first major long-term studies of healthy aging people under the auspices at the National Institutes of Health, I found that elderly people with a tendency to reminisce were regarded by many other physicians and most of society as displaying an early sign of "senile psychosis," the ailment we have come to call Alzheimer's. Today it seems an extraordinary misunderstanding, but the rather ill-informed professional consensus among authors of psychology and gerontology textbooks in the 1950s dismissed older people who engaged in reminiscing as "garrulous," "boring," and "living in the past." Their minds were "wandering," the professionals thought, with the implication that their memories were useless.

No doubt part of the explanation is that Americans have always been a forward-looking people who put great faith in progress. Yet studies done over a period of many years by me and other researchers associated with the International Longevity Center have found that reminiscences in later life have an important role, as aging people all undergo an important inner experience. The term "life review" was coined to describe this process of reminiscence, and today continuing research buttresses the importance of looking backward.

Life review can occur spontaneously, or it can be structured. The process has value for a range of ages. For any adult, in fact, but especially those in a time of transition occasioned by a career shift, the end of a marriage, or simply the desire for change, life review can offer a new perspective that can be enriching.

Dorothy's experience suggests the value of life review. A round and jolly woman in her early seventies, Dorothy has faced her share of life's challenges, including health problems (emphysema, for one) and a difficult marriage to a man whose growing deafness echoes his manner (all his life, he has heard only what he wants to hear). But she has made the best of things, and her ease with people and infectious laugh have won her many friends.

When Dorothy and her husband moved, at his insistence, to an assisted-living facility, she decided she needed a forum for making new friends. On her first Wednesday in residence, she invited several women she had just met to join her for an informal meeting; she described it as a "conversation—you know, just to talk about how we got here." Not knowing what else to talk about at the first meeting with these new acquaintances, Dorothy asked each of the women to describe an old friendship that, for whatever reason, went awry. No one was prepared for that extraordinary first session, and the tears and laughter that accompanied the stories told.

Since then Dorothy has tasked herself and the other attendees to look closely at the lives they have lived. The group has grown to more than a dozen, and Dorothy chairs their monthly meetings. The get-togethers have become a fixture in the members' lives—some of them plan their vacations so as to be around the first Wednesday of every month—and the other women value Dorothy for her ability to look at her own past (and sometimes theirs) with a critical distance that is both candid and kind. The work the women do together is, in a sense, historic, and the members of the group call themselves the Forget-Me-Nots, in recognition of the memories that should not be shunted aside. Dorothy's desire to make a few new friends has actually changed all of their lives in small but important ways.

Wrestling with Recollections

For most people, life review offers a mixture of joy and sadness, regret and satisfaction, opportunity and trepidation. It may motivate attempts at reconciliation; it may provide perspective, direction, or resolution. At a time of life when forgetfulness can be worrying, it can provide a disciplined and reassuring means of exploring one's past. I think you will find that there can be a happy sweetness about recollecting the old days.

Remembering a Life. Life review can be an individual activity, but it is often conducted in a group setting. The purpose can be an informal process of discovery or therapeutic in a more structured setting, guided by a trained psychotherapist or psychiatrist. It can be done within the embrace of a family, too, in which a grandchild or a grown child engage with a grandparent or parent to assemble a set of life recollections. Such sessions may produce happy memories but also hard ones that can lead to a useful consensus about contentious moments in the past and help the parties clarify complex family issues. Even if the parties cannot agree on their interpretations, chances are their understandings will come closer together as the process unfolds.

Asking the Questions. Whatever the circumstance, the goal is the assemblage and exploration of a life. In workshop settings, lesson plans may guide participants along a prescribed path to the past, but the areas of exploration, whatever the means, are likely to include work, marriage, childhood and parenthood, family transitions, death and loss, money, and health. Exercises can be useful in relaxing and reopening; collecting memories in journals or sharing them with others can help consolidate disparate pieces. The gist of the discussion is the fabric of a life.

Thinking Autobiography. The memoir has become a publishing phenomenon, but within families and other groups, written recollections of past events have become popular, too, a means by which individuals record recollections they value, often in order to convey what they have learned to those they love. Autobiography—a life history as recounted by the person who lived it—can be liberating and revealing. One proven approach has long been used by the widely respected gerontologist James Birren, a colleague of mine who spent more than twenty-five years enabling groups to look into their past. He published a guidebook to the process called *Telling the Stories of Life Through Guided Autobiography Groups.*

The Tools of Memory. Marcel Proust required only a small teacake (*petite madeleine*) to send him off on his immensely long trip down memory lane, *Remembrance of Things Past*, but family photo albums, scrapbooks, heirlooms, books, magazines, old movies, school yearbooks, holiday cards, or other possessions may help launch a journey of discovery. Sometimes the approach is chronological, working forward from youth through the passing years; some find it easier to access the past by working backward from the present. For others, a family history provides a useful backbone for the process.

Whatever the means of releasing locked-up memories, the result can be a valuable legacy to be shared; the inexplicable can suddenly make sense. Yet often the picture is not perfectly clear. Our memories are usually complex, nuanced, emotional, often inchoate and contradictory, and are frequently filled with irony, comedy, and tragedy.

Beware the Risks. In therapeutic sessions, life review has in some instances been a factor in the onset of depression. The risk is greater for the person who conducts the life review in isolation; individuals who are able to share the experience of the process are more likely to gain a sense of self-esteem. For some people who have carried grudges or resentments, looking at the past can provide an opportunity to even old scores or reshape events in ways that can be hurtful to others.

Life review can be a cause for genuine celebration in the very old, the old, and the aging-but-not-so-old alike. Hospice workers have found that exploring the dying person's life story can provide comfort, both to the ailing person and his or her family. Human resource professionals involved in job retraining use some of the same techniques to explore possibilities and potentials. You may wish to do the same as you think about your life. Life has moral, personal, and emotional dimensions that merit exploration as we seek to locate ourselves in our own life story, whether we near its end or are planning for the scenes to come.

Dealing with Depression

The weight of depression does more than bring spirits down. Studies have found that depression in older people actually produces memory loss. Other studies have found depression may have a causal relationship with heart disease and even cancer.

More than six million Americans age sixty-five and older are depressed. The problem is so commonplace that there is a theory among some researchers that depression is a normal part of the aging process but, in a lively and ongoing debate, others reject such thinking. Their counterhypothesis is that older people often become depressed because of physical health problems.

Many depressed people do not seek treatment, but American society has made important gains in confronting mental health issues. Not so long ago, there was a stigma attached to seeking psychiatric care, and many health insurers offered little or no coverage for treatment. Today, in contrast, there is a widespread recognition that mental illnesses of all sorts are to be regarded just as we regard physical ailments.

The aging years inevitably involve challenges, among them coping with the loss of parents and peers. Patterns of life established over decades may be disrupted by the departure of children, retirement, relocation, or illness. Change can be invigorating—but it also can produce a range of complex feelings, including sadness, fear, and a sense of being overwhelmed by bad news and negative change.

DIAGNOSING DEPRESSION. Most of us have thoughts of death as we contemplate the loss of loved ones, another birthday, illness, or even the changing seasons. Musing on one's mortality, at least occasionally, is quite normal. As the great economist John Maynard Keynes once remarked, "In the long run, we are all dead." To pretend otherwise can hardly be regarded as healthy.

On the other hand, a persistent, morbid preoccupation with death, accompanied by a sense of dread is a different matter, and may be a sign of depression. If you feel especially low, ask yourself these questions:

- Are your feelings of sadness and grief sometimes overwhelming?
- Have you lost interest in activities you used to enjoy? Have people commented on your withdrawal?
- Is your concentration poor? Are you forgetful? Do you feel indecisive at times?

- Do you have difficulty sleeping or have your sleeping patterns changed? Do you awaken early on some mornings or oversleep most days? Are you tired all the time?
- Have you gained or lost substantial weight?
- Do you feel restless and unable to sit still sometimes?
- Do you feel guilty, helpless, or worthless?
- Do you think about death or suicide?

"Yes" answers to two or more of these questions suggest you should seek the counsel of your physician or a therapist. There are people to talk to and therapies that can help you feel better, including a type of psychotherapeutic approach called cognitive behavioral therapy, which can help you change negative thinking, address problems in healthy ways, and in general cope more effectively with life's challenges.

If you feel depressed or anxious, you are not alone. Discuss the treatment options with your physician. These include mood-altering medications, psychotherapy, and other approaches such as light therapy (for seasonal depression) and electroconvulsive therapy (for severe depression). Your doctor may offer other treatments if he or she identifies an underlying cause, which can include prescription medications (some steroids, beta-blockers, anticancer agents, blood-pressure treatments, and other drugs can, in susceptible individuals, cause depression).

Do not underestimate the value of spending time with friends and family. Isolation and loneliness—often key factors in depression—may be addressed by companionship and caring. Seek out the company of those you love.

Strategy Three: Improve Your Lifestyle Choices

The task is to live a healthy lifestyle. There are proven links between maintaining mental vitality and overall physical health: Regular exercise helps maintain a good blood supply to the brain, while smoking has multiple negative impacts on the brain. Good nutrition, stress management, and other lifestyle factors have important impacts on the mind, emotions, and memory.

THE ASSIGNMENT. Now is the time to change some bad habits.

1. Select one of the action items from the following list.
2. Resolve to make the change; if you fall back one day, try again the next.
3. Keep a record. Researchers report the value of keeping a journal; individuals report that putting words to paper lowers stress, helps them quit smoking, and enables them to relax at bedtime.
4. After one month, select a second action and incorporate it into your life (do not abandon the first one). Repeat one month later and each month thereafter.

THE CHANGES. Here are some choices:

- *Quit smoking.* There are many reasons to quit, but yet another has recently been reported by the Radiological Society of North America. Researchers found that the chemical makeup of the brain is altered by smoking. Nicotine suppresses important brain chemicals, including choline, which is essential for healthy cell membranes and brain function.
- *Get enough sleep.* Insufficient sleep, plain and simple, interferes with cognitive function. Try to get eight hours of relaxing sleep per night (if you have sleeping difficulties, see *Prescription III: Seek Essential Sleep*, page 83).
- *Face down depression.* Are you depressed? If you are, seek professional care (see also *Dealing with Depression*, page 47).

- *Manage your stress levels.* Stress can destroy brain cells, so employ strategies to manage or avoid excess stress (see *Prescription IV: Set Stress Aside*, page 103).

- *Get plenty of exercise (for older people who previously have not exercised).* Moderate aerobic activity, like walking, improves function in executive tasks, such as problem solving. Walking, running, exercising at a fitness facility, dancing, and other physical activities will help keep you sharp. Do it daily, if you can (in any case, at least three times a week), and build on your current level to stay motivated. Research indicates that regular exercise is linked with a significant reduction in risk for Alzheimer's disease, dementia, and other forms of cognitive decline. (See *Prescription VI: Live the Active Life*, page 138.)

- *Employ nutritional strategies.* Never underestimate the importance of good nutrition in overall health; a healthy diet is vital to the health of your brain, too. Chose a varied mix of foods, as your body and brain need a complete range of nutrients for optimal function. A daily multivitamin or mineral supplement can help ensure that you receive the recommended daily allowance of nutrients. Research also suggests that a high-fat diet in adulthood may contribute to the risk of Alzheimer's, so the intake of fatty foods (especially those high in saturated fat) should be minimized. Eat plenty of fruit, vegetables, nuts, and seeds, as they are all high in antioxidants, which are thought to help reduce the risk of developing Alzheimer's disease. (See *Prescription VII: Eat Your Way to Health*, page 179.)

- *If you need hearing aids or new glasses, get them.* These are tools that will help in your intellectual, social, and cultural life.

- *Practice prevention.* Brain vitality cannot be separated from overall body health; cognition suffers in the presence of medical issues such as hypertension, heart disease, diabetes, high cholesterol, mini-strokes, environmental exposure to toxins such as lead and mercury, and severe head trauma.

The Old Grow Sage

Winston Churchill once observed, "We are happier in many ways when we are old than when we are young. The young sow wild oats, the old grow sage." The Nobel Prize–winning writer and British prime minister knew something of the subject: He lived to age ninety, continuing to write and paint, and he even served as a Member of Parliament until the year before his death, despite repeated strokes and a long battle with depression.

For those of us on the far side of fifty, Churchill's observation holds a certain promise: Sage (the plant) is, after all, a perennial, its leaves are flavorful, its constitution rugged. But the aphorism implies a transition, a transformation, which we all acknowledge. It is worth trying to understand that process.

A child passes through stages of development; that we accept as obvious and true. There is no general agreement as to precisely what those phases are—theorists for centuries have been formulating models to explain how we mature, from the ancient Chinese social philosopher Confucius through the father of psychoanalysis, Sigmund Freud. Other seminal thinkers have included cognitive theorist Jean Piaget, behaviorist B. F. Skinner, and educator Maria Montessori, each of whom posited various stages in our sexual, behavioral, cognitive, and social development. Some reject the notion of stages, preferring to think of change in terms of a gradual evolution rather than clear-cut transitions.

The process of adult development is even less certain than that of childhood; not so many decades ago, many experts regarded life after adolescence as little more than a long, downward journey. While no single model seems to explain the complex continuum of human development from birth to grave, a composite understanding of what is, at best, a loose consensus, may be useful as we go about considering life's vitality.

Most of us can agree that young children work to master trust, confidence, and competence as they prepare to separate from their parents. During adolescence, the youngster's identity emerges, making the person distinct and separate from his or her parents. Development surely continues, but the tasks differ in young adulthood, in midlife, and in the later years.

Freud made few allowances for adult development, as his speculations focused on sexual development in childhood and adolescence. But a next-generation follower, Erik Erikson, saw growth and development as a lifelong psychosocial cycle. Developing upon the work of Erikson and others, a collective understanding has emerged that suggests that as a young adult, the chief developmental imperative becomes learning how to manage a new kind of bond with another person. This intimacy makes healthy relationships possible, partnerships that are not self-centered but are shared. In middle adulthood, the desire to nurture emerges, and may be employed in raising children or creating change that benefits other people in a family or in a working environment or both.

In these pages, we are more interested in what follows thereafter.

As Erikson saw it, the next stage is characterized by a tension between what he called *generativity* and *stagnation*. He saw resolving this as the work of the middle adult years (roughly ages thirty-five to sixty-five). Erikson identified the desire for fulfilling and creative work and the wish to be useful (perhaps by marriage and child-rearing) as generativity. In short, we derive strength from caring for others and transmitting our values within a stable environment of our creation; that's the generative part. Failure to act upon that instinct, on the other hand, will result in stagnation. With the departure of our children we face a risk of self-absorption as we look for new purposes and meanings.

As people in the twenty-first century age and remain remarkably healthy into their sixties, seventies, and beyond, the importance of generativity does not disappear at age sixty or seventy or even eighty. As the need for achievement decreases, a rich sense of fulfillment can be gained from community work, teaching, mentoring, and other ways of guiding younger people. Generativity involves a paradoxical capacity for leadership (age can confer a certain authority) and yet a willingness to forgo the kind of control a parent exercises over a child in favor of a respect for autonomy. Call it empathic leadership, if you will, but as one recent book, *Aging Well*, by George E. Vaillant, M.D., pointed out, people who master generativity *triple* the chances that the decade of the seventies will be a time of joy, not despair.

In Erikson's eighth and final developmental stage (he termed it *integrity vs. despair*), the human animal takes a retrospective look back over the decades of his or her life. In late adulthood, those who feel contentment, happiness, and fulfillment when they regard their earlier years, a sense of achievement or meaning may coalesce; Erikson called that feeling of a life well spent *integrity*. If the outlook is not so positive, if the sensation is one of doubt or gloom, then the perceived failures and the lack of a life's purpose fulfilled may produce the *despair* Erikson talks about.

Erikson's model is not universally accepted. Other writers describe the stages differently (*memory keeping* is one identifying label some people use for the valuable role an older person can play in a community or a family, which also contributes to the aging person's sense of self). In his recent book, *The Mature Mind,* Gene D. Cohen, who founded the Center on Aging at the National Institute of Mental Health, writes of developmental intelligence, which he describes as a "maturing synergy of cognition, emotional intelligence, judgment, social skills, life experience, and consciousness." Moving beyond Erikson's theory, Cohen suggests that there are four phases of psychological development in mature life, including midlife reevaluation ("a time of exploration and transition"); liberation, with its consequent desire to experiment; the summing-up phase ("recapitulation, resolution, and review"); and, finally, the "encore." To Cohen, age sixty-five does not imply retiring from life but a time of creativity, intellectual growth, and more satisfying relationships.

YOUR THREE STRATEGIES TO MENTAL VITALITY

At the core of this chapter is a three-step prescription; it requires a commitment of time and concentration. The promise is a more vital life. To review:

Strategy One: Cognitive Calisthenics

What enjoyable activity have you chosen to exercise the reserve capacity of your brain and its ability to integrate newly acquired knowledge? To review the ways in which you can put the circuitry in your brain to use, see page 26.

Strategy Two: Reconfigure Your Brain

Have you found a new way of regularly connecting with other people that takes you out of old patterns? Such activities will make you more vital— amazingly enough, some researchers have found in animal studies that intellectual stimulation actually promotes brain *growth*. For suggestions, see page 40.

Strategy Three: Improve Your Lifestyle Choices

Everyone has bad habits: Have you made a plan for correcting one or more of yours? Smoking cessation, weight control, an exercise plan ... there are many options (see page 49).

There is no one path to brain health, but in evidence-based studies the approaches cited here have been demonstrated to be effective in keeping people vital and feeling younger.

Simply looking at your life with a fresh perspective can offer a valuable challenge. The intellect, the emotions, perhaps even your spirit may benefit from such self-examination as you assess how best to spend your time, to live well and age well.

On the other hand, the aging years can be overrated and do pose challenges. Retirement, for example, may, in anticipation, seem like a dream to be fulfilled. However, many people do not realize that the workplace is their major source of intellectual and social stimulation; the loss of that day-to-day exposure to conversation, ideas, and challenges needs to be filled by other activities. By all means, retire from your day job if you wish; but do so with an awareness that you will have not only hours to fill, but you may feel a loss of purpose, structure, and companionship. Keep in mind you can un-retire if you wish. The aging years require flexibility, a willingness to adapt, and the discipline to find what you need.

Aging is not a one-way trip to senility: The momentary inability to remember the capital of North Dakota (it is Bismarck) does not signal imminent memory collapse. Cognitive function in the aging years can be thought of as resembling a network of streams running down a hillside. Call it a babbling brook, one that, over a period time, sees its course change. But be patient. As is obvious from the rising tide of articles in the scientific literature (including a comprehensive one in 2008 in the *Proceedings of National Academy of Science*), people who are willing to invest disciplined time and energy in enhancing their vitality will be rewarded by improvements in fluid intelligence and, in particular, in the performance of working memory.

PRESCRIPTION II

NURTURE YOUR RELATIONSHIPS

❖

WE KNOW INTUITIVELY THAT A WARM SENSE OF CONNECTEDNESS to others helps make us human. More surprising is that, according to a growing body of research, a sense of belonging also keeps us healthy.

The life-giving importance of human contact was observed long ago in newborns. Quite simply, a tiny baby must be touched to feel secure. In the absence of loving contact and the accompanying sense of nurture, babies tend to slip into a syndrome called "failure to thrive" in which they develop slowly, their stress levels soar, and, as adults very much later, they are more likely to have social problems.

In adults, it is much the same: To thrive throughout life, we benefit from attachments, whether you call it love, friendship, empathy, or bonding. Those connections can add great richness to the three-decade dividend.

To get specific: Over the last decade a series of published studies has found that people in happy marriages are less likely to suffer from heart disease than those in unhappy marriages or who are divorced or widowed. According to a national longitudinal study (a longitudinal study looks at a group over an extended period), it is true in men; more recently (the results were published in 2005) the finding was affirmed in women, too.

Other ongoing studies are enlarging our understanding of the phenomenon. The instinct for reciprocal, caring connection comes to inform a range of relationships beyond parent and young child and the intimacies of spouses and partners. It is echoed in the special link between siblings, the confiding ties of friendship, the pleasures of a soul mate, and the extraordinary challenges and satisfactions posed by the parent-child bond. In these relationships, individuals are enriched by ties to others in conscious and subconscious ways.

In this chapter, the focus will be on loved ones but, to be clear, I will define our terms. A loved one might be a spouse, one of your children, a sibling, a parent, or a grandparent. Intimate friends, a trusted coworker, and a neighbor might belong here, too. These are the people who *know* us, the ones we truly know. Central to this chapter will be our life partners, the individuals with whom we have paired ourselves for the long term; necessarily, then, the physical intimacy we share with our spouse, lover, or partner fits here, too, so sexuality is discussed in the pages to come. In a later chapter, *Prescription V: Connect with Your Community*, I will talk of the arm's length universe of people, many of whom we may like very much but to whom we are unlikely to confide our secrets (see page 120). In that chapter you will find other important relationships, but here the subject is the immediate and elemental connection with our loved ones.

You must cherish them as they cherish you. They are the ones who give us reason to live.

WHEN SHE WAS IN HER LATE SEVENTIES, Elizabeth Pond fell while working in her garden and broke a hip. Two days later, her surgeon performed a hip arthroplasty, and within a week she was released from the hospital.

She confided in her son (one of my colleagues) that she was very glad to be home. "I couldn't have been away any longer. I knew your father was running out of clean dishes and the kitchen would be a hopeless mess." She said it with a straight face and her usual directness. She was not kidding. She knew that, after more than fifty years of marriage, she had a range of responsibilities and a life she wanted to resume living.

Some years later, however, she fell again and broke her other hip. By then she was a widow, living in an assisted-living facility, and experiencing the mental fog that accompanies the early stages of Alzheimer's disease. She would never walk unassisted again; she died only a few months later. A big factor, her physician told her son, was that this time there was no get-well imperative. The doctor knew that she was physically capable of making a strong recovery, but the changes in her world had left her with no target to aim for, no reason to live.

The story has a sad ending, but a bigger piece of the story is the strong marriage that Elizabeth enjoyed for fifty-nine years.

do not be embarrassed to embrace

The health-giving properties of human contact may seem an intangible, but its effects have actually been measured. Consider the study reported in 2003 by Karen Grewen and Kathleen Light, two psychology professors at the University of North Carolina at Chapel Hill.

The researchers assembled two mixed groups of some ninety couples, men and women who were married or living together. After taking baseline readings of each individual's heart rate and blood pressure, the investigators encouraged members of the first group to hold hands as they watched a ten-minute romantic video, then to embrace for twenty seconds afterward. In comparison to this "warm-contact" group, the couples in the control group simply sat together for a period of ten minutes and twenty seconds. All the couples were then asked to speak to a group of people about a personal experience that caused them to feel stress or anger, during which blood pressure and heart rate were monitored. The results were striking: The stress of speaking to the group produced an increase in blood pressure and heart rate across the board—but the increases were consistently less among members of the warm-contact group. The effect was measurably greater among the roughly a third of the participants who were African-American.

The lesson? The findings clearly suggest that an affectionate relationship with a supportive partner can lessen the stress of facing life events; the researchers, in fact, concluded that the benefit of marital support may produce better overall cardiovascular health.

Life can be busy, the tide of events so powerful, that we forget the small things. These minor moments and taken-for-granted gestures are surprisingly important. We can, and perhaps should, share them with our loved ones. So do not underestimate the value of touching, hugging, and sharing in the face of life's nonstop demands.

The Supportive Life

As a physician, I find it gratifying—and a little surprising—that it is a statistical fact that a good marriage at age fifty is a better predictor of good health at age eighty than a low cholesterol count. The life-enhancing power of marriage is further evidence that, quite simply, individuals of the species thrive on shared, generous, reassuring, interdependent, friendly, and loving interactions with other members of the human race (whether or not, it should be said, the bond has been officially sanctioned by church or state).

The supportive life reaches well beyond the bounds of our connections to life partners. In fact, we can take the strength of intimacy a step further: Most professionals in the longevity field accept the general notion that love lengthens life. Not simply the physical act of love (although sexual intimacy may play a role, too). Rather, we are talking about that most powerful of human emotions, the selfless commitment and caring that we feel for our loved ones, our communities, and even our world.

As we mature, one essential capacity we develop is the natural give-and-take of friendship. As life's demands begin to lessen during the aging years, our need for others with whom to share our feelings, insights, and beliefs can increase. The idealized notions of the happily-ever-after of Hollywood's celluloid dreams have faded a bit; we are wiser in some ways, perhaps, but no less desirous of friendship in an inclusive sense. Your spouse can be your friend, but so can the classmate you meet up with at your fiftieth reunion and with whom, despite not exchanging a word in decades, you find you continue to share the same sense of humor or pathos about life.

It is a practical and emotional reality that most of us function better when we have friendships we can rely upon. How important are friends? Researchers have found that happiness tends to be greater for those with lots of friendships than those with few worries about retirement income. I will put it more bluntly: Friendship is priceless.

The ability to make friends is an attribute some people simply seem to have, like big feet or red hair. Just ask the lonely preschooler. Yet making and keeping friends is not an effortless enterprise for anyone, even if, at times, it appears that way.

Friendship is a skill, one that grows in importance with the passing years. As a man who has outlived a beloved wife and many friends, I understand that when we lose a friend, there is a hole to fill. We are not general managers concerned with filling the roster on a ball team; it is more complicated than that. Friendship is a blend of liking, respect, and trust; and it's reciprocal, too, since for a friendship to endure those feelings must go both ways.

Family is another key component of the supportive life. There are great joys in a range of family relationships—but, once again, none is automatic. You need to be prepared to reach out, to let your children, grandchildren, and other relations know that the door is open.

Some happy familial relationships seem to evolve naturally, but to maintain others you may need to find new ways to relate. Often when our children mature and embark on their own lives, our relationships with them undergo a sea change. They need independence and we need to respect that, but as the years pass, I have observed that many are happy to drift back into a new version of that old and special parent-child relationship. A process of redefinition may already have taken place, but if it has not, go slowly and make no presumptions. This is a new sort of friendship you are shaping; it needs to be mutual like any other.

Try to see things from their perspective (empathy, the ability to understand another person's feelings or difficulties, is invaluable at any age). Ask about their lives and concerns. Make a mental note of what it is they are worried about or hoping for, following up at an appropriate time (*Whatever happened with . . . ?*). If you're genuinely interested in them, they are much more likely to be interested in you.

With grandchildren, find activities in common. It may be tennis or golf on a Wii, the electronic gaming device that allows you to mimic the moves of sports and compete with others from the comfort of your home. It could be shopping, the county fair, a movie, a TV show you can share. Or you can take a trip—for an afternoon, a weekend, or longer to celebrate an anniversary or other event with the whole family.

Nurture—the tender care we give to a growing child—has a key place in the way we regard people we love, whether friends or family. Caring and time invested can nurture these important connections.

LONGEVITY AWARENESS CHECK

Ask yourself these questions:

Q: *When was the last time you embraced someone out of sheer affection rather than social convention?*

Q: *The last time you felt a twinge of longing to talk to a long-lost friend or relative, did you act upon it?*

Q: *How long has it been since you last apologized for hurting someone's feelings, even if it wasn't intentional?*

Q: *Are you involved in a relationship in which you share mutually satisfying sexual intimacies?*

Q: *Is the giving and receiving of human affection a normal part of your life?*

The vital life involves regular and meaningful contact with friends, family, and others.

Strategy Four: Maintaining Friendships

The task is to enhance your caring connections. Like most everything of a certain age, friendships are subject to the wear and tear of time. Their vintage often tends to enrich and deepen them (like fine wine or the patina on a piece of fine furniture), but friendships also require appropriate care and maintenance.

THE ASSIGNMENT. My recommendation is that you seek ways to nurture your friendships. Try this:

1. Begin by identifying three friendships that are important to you.
2. Pick one that is healthy and active; select another that has gone dormant for no particular reason; choose a third that was broken at some point in the past.
3. Examine all three for lessons good and bad, and try to put all of them in good working order.

FRIENDLY BEHAVIORS. Here are some ways to enhance your friendships:

- *Remember that friends listen.* When you need to vent anger, share a sorrow, worry a decision, confide a secret fear or hope, or just talk something through, the good friend lends an ear. In return, though, you are on call to do the same. The sensitive friend knows whether the task at hand is merely to listen or to offer advice or constructive criticism. Use the common experience as a basis, but do not take it for granted.
- *Be conscious of change.* Sensitivity to the shifting sands of friendship is invaluable. It is not a given that the bonds of yesteryear are unchanging. When a friend's world is shaken—death, chronic disease,

divorce, alcoholism, job loss, a doted-upon child moving across the country—try on your friend's shoes for a moment to see how they feel. Even if the change is less radical, be sensitive.

- *Think before you speak.* Words that belittle others do not make you better, bigger, and smarter. Honesty is to be valued, but there is almost always a way to be candid *and* kind. Even if you feel the weight of truth, morality, or wisdom is on your side, take your friend's priorities into consideration. Even if you are utterly certain about something—who the better candidate is in an election, for example—your friend may not share your opinion. Do not presume you know better.

- *Know your audience.* Distinguish between what *you* think is a fascinating story and what actually engages other people's interest. You may wish to share your joy in a story, but are you actually just enjoying the sound of your own voice? Know the difference.

- *Friends first.* Even with old friends, do not forget to inquire into their lives. Ask them about themselves, rather than just telling them about yourself. Listen with care to criticisms offered by others, too.

- *Practice forgiveness.* I have heard the term "Irish Alzheimer's." It describes the condition—common in all demographics—in which a person forgets everything but the grudge. A much healthier approach is a two-stage process: First you forgive, then you forget. Anger, especially simmering anger, is a powder keg ready for the spark. Talk it through, work it through.

- *Deal with estrangements.* Some friendships end quietly, like a power cord disconnected from a wall socket; some end with a flash of emotional lighting and a thunderclap. If you have disconnections in your past, consider why. It is very possible that the original cause is now outweighed by other needs; if you have forgotten the details of the disagreement, the difference probably has ceased to be important. Make amends and apologies. It won't hurt.

- *Be positive.* You do not have to play Pollyanna and see the world only in rosy hues. On the other hand, always seeing the dark clouds is neither good for you nor fun for your friends.

- *Do not be presidential.* Even if you are accustomed to running things, do not think you are in charge of every friendship or exchange.

- *Loving yourself is essential.* Only if you respect and appreciate yourself can you establish and maintain healthy relationships with others.

- *Saying no is okay.* If there are times when you feel as if you are always doing other people's bidding, you should sometimes say *No!* Being taken for granted is diminishing.

- *Try out tolerance.* Think of it like buying a shirt or blouse in a pattern that is not ordinarily your style: Identify a person or group that you distrust or dislike and work to change your attitude. The human body and our mental attitudes tend to stiffen a bit with time; try out a little flexibility. Think of it as emotional elasticity.

- *Practice self-discipline.* Follow up on a resolution you have held in abeyance: Quit smoking or start that walking regime, for example. Small accomplishments add up to a stronger sense of self. Feeling better about yourself may make you a better friend, too.

- *Express your feelings.* If it feels like you should, tell people you love them or that you value their company, that you are happy to see them.

- *Do not be smothering.* Express yourself, but also be sensitive to and respectful of other people's boundaries.

- *Be accessible.* Even if you have sworn never to own one, get a cell phone. You'll find it makes staying in touch easier, and the prices are no longer prohibitive. As long as you don't use it when driving, it can be considered a safety tool, too, for emergencies and quick response. Sending a text message on your phone is surprisingly easy; such messages are a means of reminding people you are there without demanding time or talk in return.

- *Try acceptance.* Just as you are independent and self-sufficient, you need to give your friends the space they need.
- *Keep in touch.* Make an effort to see people: Even if it is no more than a phone call or an e-mail, keep in contact.
- *Feed your friends.* A meal, a lunch, a pie, or some other eating opportunity almost always sets the right tone for an interaction.
- *Consider your consumption.* What may seem like lighthearted social drinking can become alcohol abuse over time. Researchers have found that alcohol abuse is a key predictor of problems in the aging years. The problem drinker often loses friends, becomes isolated, and his or her social support systems erode. For men who consume more than two alcoholic drinks a day, for women who consume more than one daily, and anyone who binge drinks (defined as five drinks or more), alcohol is a looming problem. Seek help. (See *Alcohol: Tonic or Toxin?* on page 193.)

TIME CAN BE A MEASURE of friendship. Despite all the changes that the years bring—geographic distance, educational differences, marital transitions, the coming and going of children—some friendships endure. Even at a remove from the shared circumstances that originally brought people together, a common bond can survive and grow.

Sara, Thelma, Sue, and Marybeth met when they were preadolescent girls summering on New Hampshire's Lake Winnipesaukee. That was back in the years just after World War II. Even then they hailed from different places, including suburban Boston, New York City, and industrial New Jersey. But they shared the emotional roller coaster ride that is the teen years—boys, schools, parents, and the biological, intellectual, and emotional transitions of growing up.

In their middle seventies now, all four women (and their husbands) are retired, and, for most of the year, they live in Honolulu, Los Angeles, Gulf Coast Florida, and eastern Massachusetts. But for the summer months, their lives are still based around a freshwater cove on New Hampshire's biggest lake, where they all reside in the same simple summer cottages they knew as schoolgirls.

Their connection wasn't unbroken; military service, parenting, divorce, health problems, and other life events kept each of them away from Winnipesaukee for long periods. However, for the last twenty years, they have had a "walking friendship" that has reawakened and sustained their earlier connections. On non-rainy mornings, they meet at 7:30 and walk together. It is not a power walk, though the purpose is partly exercise, and they follow more or less the same route. As they walk, they talk about everything. As Sara describes their morning ritual, "Our talks each morning are often mundane and frequently silly, but there is real intimacy there as well. We can get to the heart of any matter quickly, as we know each other's history and the cast of characters so well. Friendships that have continuity and opportunity are rare," she adds, "and because we do not see each other for seven months of the year, we truly appreciate it."

Strategy Five: Making New Friends

The dislocations that come with time, whether the cause is divorce, death, or retirement, can mean a sense of isolation and loneliness. Finding friends can alter the landscape, but making friends requires a real desire to be one.

THE ASSIGNMENT. My prescription is to invite new people into your life. To do that, attempt the following:

1. Look at and into yourself with an eye to improving your skills at negotiating the terrain of friend-making.
2. Find opportunities to make new acquaintances that, over time, may be nurtured into friends.

THE APPROACHES. As you seek to broaden your circle, here are some techniques to help you:

- *Decide what you desire in a friend.* This is a key question to ponder. Among the likely attributes is trust. A priority may be a person who shares your sense of humor or likes to read or go to the movies. Good friends are curious and caring, patient, nonjudgmental, and do not take advantage. They do not burden one another. Being a good friend is not so different from a being a good scout: A Boy Scout is taught that he should be trustworthy, loyal, helpful, friendly, courteous, kind, cheerful, thrifty, clean, and prepared, and that he ought to do a good turn daily. Does that sound like you? If it does not, think about how you could change to fit the description. What you desire in a friend probably is very similar to what a potential friend will want to see in you.
- *Update your attitudes.* Still think a woman is not supposed to call a man? Think again. That rule is changing; if you want to make a new friend, make the call.
- *Go out into the world.* Attend events in your community that interest you. If you enjoy the theater, party politics, poetry readings, or sporting events, you probably will find like-minded people to talk to at gatherings of such interest groups. One conversation can lead to another, one meeting to a second.
- *Find groups to join.* Church groups, community groups, and clubs are good opportunities; common ground is often fertile ground for friendship. If you have a social or health issue in your life, sup-

port groups may expose you to other people facing the same challenges, as well as to strategies for dealing with a particular disease or illness (arthritis, alcoholism, cancer, and a range of other life challenges often are the basis of community or hospital-based organizations).

- *Take a trip.* Go on cruise. Take a bus tour. Attend that reunion.
- *Don't forget e-mail.* E-mail has become an easy means of keeping in contact with new friends and old.
- *Communicate.* Communication is at the core of all healthy relationships. Many means are available, some as nonintrusive as "texting" (sending a text messaging from your cell phone to someone else's, just a few words of greeting or to share a fun fact). New or old, the good rules of maintaining friendships still apply (see *Strategy Four: Maintaining Friendships*, page 63).
- *Let go of greed and need.* If age brings wisdom, one of its most valuable lessons concerns the lust for money and power. The yearning to succeed and to accumulate money and worldly things is almost a given among the young; the ability to channel those desires in ways that are individually and socially constructive develops with time. Not only is the old cliché true (You can't take it with you), but it can be valuable in encountering the world with less greed and more of a sense of its needs.
- *Stow the stoicism.* Gentlemen, I am talking mostly to you: Try listening to your inner minds and spirits sometimes, instead of pretending you are not hearing the voice.
- *Reconnect.* Your college roommate? A long-lost cousin? There are many means—technological, telephonic, and old-fashioned networking—of finding the whereabouts of people you remember fondly from the past. Try alumni listings and Internet searches; a blind e-mail may lead to something important. An old friend made new can bring the dual pleasures of discovery and recollection.

Sexuality

Sexuality is important during the reproductive years—the survival of the species depends upon it—but, for most of us, shared physical intimacies are also integral to our overall health and quality of life for many years thereafter. Our sexuality does not simply vanish at menopause, be it the male or female variety, but remains part of our individual identities. For the vast majority of us, the capacity for sexual expression outlives the reproductive capability and, often, lasts throughout the dividend decades.

Sex is far from simple, whatever our age. It serves a reproductive purpose, of course, which in itself is an immensely complex process. But sexuality is actually an elegant and highly integrated system of biophysiological, psychological, and social functions. I have studied and written about sexuality in the past, and the more I learn about sexuality, the more evident it is to me that our sexual behaviors provide perhaps the most tangible evidence for mind-body interconnectedness, a linkage between our brains and our bodies that may explain more about our overall health than traditional medicine once realized.

Despite the role that sexuality continues to play in our lives throughout the life course, frank discussion concerning problems, preferences, disease, and even the importance of sexuality in the aging years is far from usual. Ironically, we live in world where a massive sexual marketplace thrives (ten years ago would you have supposed that the term "erectile dysfunction" would become a familiar epithet to everyone who watches television?), yet open discussion of sex and intimacy in some quarters remains censored by religion or politics.

That has begun to change, as has the once widely held assumption that older people simply lose interest in sex. Perhaps Supreme Court Chief Justice Oliver Wendell Holmes had it about right. Not only did he serve on the Court until age ninety (three cheers for longevity and the lively mind!), but Justice Holmes remained available to other stimuli, too. As Holmes once said upon watching a pretty girl walk by, "Oh, to be eighty again!"

AM I TOO OLD FOR SEX? A study published in 2007 in the *New England Journal of Medicine* reported that not only sexual desire but also the ability to act upon it is by no means merely a memory for most people in their aging years. Investigators found that *three-quarters* of the Americans in the nationally representative sample remain sexually active in the decade before their sixty-fifth birthday, and that *more than half* continued to have sexual relations with a partner in the next decade. Despite a significant increase in health problems, the loss of partners, and other factors, *more than a quarter* of those surveyed who were age seventy-five and older still reported active sex lives.

Lucky are those who, after fifty years of marriage, can report that they are living with their best friend. Yet surveys encounter this reaction with surprising frequency; almost as often, interviewers are also told that these couples' sex lives remain regular and satisfying.

A small minority of adults do choose celibacy (abstinence from sex), and the physical component of love as we express it through sexuality fluctuates through life. The passing of years can have an impact on your sex life. For men, the production of testosterone tends to fall and erectile difficulties to increase; for women the physiological changes that accompany menopause may produce a number of changes, ranging from vaginal dryness to diminished desire. For many people, however, these prove to be minor impediments and the practice of intimacy—physical and emotional connectedness—for many older people continues to be pleasurable, rewarding, and fulfilling.

⁜

VIRGINIA WAS A WIDOW of eighty-one when she met Mr. James. He had been a dance instructor until two years before, when, upon turning eighty, he gifted his son the studio and retired. But he was still spry when Virginia met him through mutual friends. Although her Texas drawl contrasted with his Brooklyn accent, the two found each other to be very good company.

Virginia's son began to worry as his mother and her gentleman caller began spending more and more time together. One Saturday night he dropped by at her apartment unexpectedly and found the two eightysomethings *dancing*! He was outraged and told his mother so. She laughed off his concern, but he was mortified.

Her daughter-in-law, Martha, recognized what her son did not: Virginia, after having been trapped in an unhappy marriage for almost fifty years, was delighted with the attention, company, and good humor of the sociable Mr. James. When Virginia confided that she and Mr. James were talking of marriage, Martha was thrilled, but her husband was soon grumbling about his mother giving away the family name ("It is not *her* name," Martha reminded him). But he was mollified when his mother told him there was not going to be "any of that sex stuff." Privately, Virginia told Martha, she had lied a little, just to relieve her son. "It's different now," she confided with a shy smile.

Sexual pleasure is not sole province of the young, no matter what Virginia's son wanted to think.

THE SECOND LANGUAGE OF SEX. At the blush of early maturity, we enjoy the first language of sex. When we are young, sexual union tends to be urgent and explosive; it involves physical pleasure and, in many cases, leads to the conception of children. It is biological, instinctive, exciting, and energizing. It is a means of asserting independence, strength, prowess, and power.

As we age, however, we begin to understand as the young cannot that sex is not merely a matter of athleticism and productivity. Sexuality has a powerful emotional component; it is communicative as well as physical. It is later in life that we reach a deeper understanding of this "second language" of sex.

The second language is learned rather than instinctual. It involves a sensitivity to feelings—yours and your partner's—and an ability to share those feelings in actions, words, and perceptions. It requires that old irritations be banished. It may involve humor—since sexuality does not have to be deadly serious, there is room for smiles and laughter. Playfulness has its place, just as passion does. Giving is as crucial as getting; there are satisfactions in partnership.

The second language implies the possibility of renewal instead of routine. Experience brings appreciation; sexuality represents not only youth but self-discovery, skill, change, and perspective.

Most of all, it expresses the reciprocal love we can share with another person. You undoubtedly understand something of sexuality's second language; if you work on it, your abilities to speak this language will improve.

Adjusting to Change

Traditionally, society has seen older people as asexual. When we were young, many of us simply assumed that to be old was to be no longer interested (or capable). Society was content to believe that people inhabited their "golden years" as old, worn out, and disinterested in sex.

I think we can agree that much has changed. With the demographic explosion of longevity, more people are living much longer, and many more of them regard themselves as sexual beings way beyond age fifty, sixty, and seventy. Sexual activity is far from unheard of in the eighties and even nineties. For some people, the sex-is-beyond-me profile still fits, but for most of us, such notions are offensive and ageist (ageism being the systematic discrimination against people because they are old).

The first adjustment, then, is to accept an image of yourself, in your own mind: You can choose to regard yourself as a sexual being, or—and this, certainly, is the choice of some—you can elect to regard sexuality as the province of the younger you or younger people. The decision is yours to make; you should not merely accept the categorization of the people around you. Even sons or daughters, love you as they do, may still think of you as they did as children; they continue to see you as parents, to deny your sexuality out of some primitive childhood need instead of accepting you as fellow adults with perfectly normal sexual needs and desires.

FEMALE SEXUALITY. In women, the most significant physiological change of later life is menopause, also called the climacteric or the "change of life."

This physiological shift usually occurs between ages forty-five and fifty-five. The signal change is the cessation of menstruation; the underlying cause is the drop in estrogen levels to about 20 percent of midlife levels. The short-term consequences often include hot flashes, fatigue, headaches, and feelings of emotional instability. Later, the bone thinning of osteoporosis can develop, in part because of the drop in estrogen levels in the body.

Postmenopausal women may experience some changes in their sexual functioning. The reduction in estrogen can mean less vaginal lubrication or a thinning of the vaginal lining. The dryness may result in a roughened texture and pain, while the thinner lining may be easily irritated and can bleed and crack. Vaginal lubricants are often very useful in decreasing or eliminating such discomforts. Be sure to use oil-based lubricants (K-Y Jelly, Astroglide, and Ortho Personal Lubricants are among the many choices) and avoid oil-based products like petroleum jelly, baby oil, and mineral oil because they do not dissolve in water and thus can facilitate vaginal infection. Hormone replacement therapy has also been proven effective (see *Hormone Replacement Therapy*, page 75).

If you experience vaginal pain or signs of infection, you should discuss the symptoms with your physician. The doctor may be able to offer some help in relieving the discomfort and will also determine whether the cause is another condition that requires treatment. Other causes may include allergies, dermatitis, bladder inflammation, cystitis, or tumors.

It is intriguing to note that there is some evidence that regular sexual activity helps maintain the vagina's ability to lubricate itself and may even stimulate the production of estrogen.

Aside from the effects of estrogen loss after menopause, normal aging appears to interfere very little with a woman's sexual ability. Other factors, however, may impact her sex life, most prominently the health status of her partner (or the absence of one). Disease, physical disability, medications, surgery, alcoholism, and tobacco use can lessen sexual desire and sexual response in men and women alike.

hormone replacement therapy

To use HRT or not? For the woman who is facing menopause, the answer is not always clear. A little history may be helpful in framing that decision.

In the late 1940s, estrogen replacement therapy came into use to treat the discomforts of menopause. The drug regimen worked; such symptoms as hot flashes, backache, lowered sex drive, and memory loss were significantly reduced. Then, in the middle seventies, ERT was linked to an increased risk of endometrial cancer (a malignancy of the lining of the uterus).

Soon a new formulation was marketed that added progestin (a synthetic form of the female hormone progesterone), which allowed the dosage of estrogen to be decreased. Effective in treating the discomforts of menopause, HRT was also credited with delivering some protection against future heart disease and osteoporosis. However, a possible link was subsequently identified between HRT use and the development of breast and ovarian cancer.

What's the menopausal woman to do? Given that HRT has clear benefits but also evident potential risks, the decision is an individual one, and should be made in consultation with your doctor. Some women experience more intense discomforts (night sweats, vaginal pain, insomnia, and even depression), while others find menopause less difficult. Your degree of discomfort may be a determinant in your decision. Some women probably should avoid HRT, especially those with a personal or family history of cancer, diabetes, blood clots, liver disease, abnormal genital bleeding, severe varicose veins, very high blood pressure, or high blood triglycerides. For those who opt for hormone replacement therapy, low doses and short-term use are recommended.

MALE SEXUALITY. Many men experience sexual changes as they age. For example, it is not uncommon for a man engaged in sexual intercourse to find the momentum toward orgasm ebbs; nothing in particular happens to cause it, but the usual rising urge may vanish from time to time. There may be underlying causes—some disease states and the overconsumption of alcohol can be causes—but changes in sexual function with age are to be expected. If it happens, you may wish to consult a physician; the doctor may ask a series of questions and even do tests and exams. But if everything is otherwise normal, the man who sometimes stops short of reaching orgasm need not feel diminished.

With the passing years, this and other changes are to be expected. The speed at which a man experiences erection will slow somewhat; it is entirely normal for some minutes to be required rather than the seconds in which his younger self responded to sexual stimulation. The erection may also be less rigid and smaller than in youth. Once excited, however, the erection is typically quite up to the task of a sexual encounter. To promote and maintain arousal, manual stimulation of the penis may be required.

There are certain advantages to the aging male sex organs. The volume of seminal fluid ejaculated decreases in the aging years, which also means the ejaculatory pressure is lessened. The older man can make love longer by delaying ejaculation. Some men also find that sex is no longer defined by ejaculation; they may have intercourse without producing sperm every time or, in some cases, at all, yet experience a sustained state of sexual pleasure and intimacy.

Strategy Six:
Maintaining Sexual Communication

Sex is one of life's pleasures. Except, of course, when it is not and, instead, it is a source of anxiety, guilt, conflict, or other unwanted feelings. Often such difficulties can be resolved, sometimes in conjunction with your partner, at times with your physician, or even a therapist. What follows is a short list of considerations that may interfere with—or enhance—the pleasures of sex—together with a few facts and suggestions to help you.

THE ASSIGNMENT. Strive to communicate better with your partner: about changes, about needs, about desires. Not all of these exchanges will be verbal; some are physical, matters of touching (or not).

SEXUAL CONCERNS. As you age, as you work through relationship and sexual difficulties, I recommend you keep the following matters in mind.

- *Anticipate variations in intimacy.* Over time, our needs change; sexual anxiety is not the sole province of the young and inexperienced. If you can ask, demur, and express yourself, your partner can, too. Shared concerns may emerge; adaptation is necessary. You may find opening up lines of communication is actually liberating for both of you; on the other hand, do not expect immediate acceptance of change.
- *Think about it as a two-way street.* Communication must go both ways. It is about *we*, not just *me*.
- *Sex and recovery.* After a heart attack or bypass surgery, sex may suddenly seem dangerous. For most people, though, the fear passes and sexual activity can resume (remember that, as a general rule, physical exercise—of which sex is one kind—leads to *less* likelihood of heart attack). Arthritis, back problems, and other health problems can make sex more difficult, but in most cases, a partnership approach that relies upon kind but clear communication can help resolve many difficulties and make satisfying sex possible.
- *Candor counts.* Be frank in telling your partner what is pleasurable and what is not, which positions are comfortable and which are not. The language of sexuality is often nonverbal: Be attuned to mood, energy levels, reluctance, and hunger. Listening is essential.
- *Be adaptable.* With the bodily changes of menopause, the use of a vaginal lubricant may be required, often in advance of having intercourse. Anticipation can help with arousal, too. A woman who drinks water and who urinates before and after intercourse may avoid cystitis, in which the bladder becomes inflamed.
- *Know about erectile dysfunction.* Almost every man sometimes doubts

his sexual potency; in fact, erectile difficulties occur at some point among virtually all men. The cause may be fatigue, tension, excessive alcohol consumption, or illness. So do not conclude your sex life is over if you experience one performance failure.

- *Sex is in your head as well as your loins.* Emotions like depression, anger, fear, and anxiety can interfere with sexual behavior. Stress in other areas of your life, your partner's disinterest, or dissatisfaction with your aging appearance can undermine desire and confidence. Both men and women experience a loss of desire as a result of life events such as retirement, illness, and the death of loved ones. Our society remains ambivalent about sex, and some older people can pick up younger people's disapproval of their sexual interest.

- *Sex is more than intercourse.* Sexual expression is, in a sense, a different means of communicating with your partner. Using your shared experience can help you achieve a level of satisfaction that is both sexual and simply companionable.

- *Self-stimulation is permitted.* Does it need to be said again? Self-stimulation is healthy: Neither blindness nor venereal disease will result from masturbation.

Sexual Dysfunction

S . . . E . . . X. The word is a mere three letters long, but it has as many meanings as there are people. Not only is every individual's sexuality distinct from everyone else's, but over time, as we pass through the stages of adolescence, early adulthood, child-bearing and the parenting years, and beyond, the expression, experience, and the meaning of sexuality fluctuates.

Sexuality is dynamic; it varies over time with age, health, relationship status, and other factors. That is all entirely normal. A gradual diminution in sexual interest and activity in the aging years is also common, but the notion that people of a certain age become asexual simply is not true. Sexual function does not inevitably wane, deteriorate, and disappear with added years. As we saw earlier in the chapter, the research suggests that sexuality continues to be a pleasure for many people well into the later decades of life.

I am not proposing that sex remains the same throughout life. In men, for example, as testosterone levels decline, the sexual response cycle more closely resembles that of women, with a prolonged phase of excitement and greater need for stimulation and foreplay. Unfortunately, many men, unaware of these normal changes in body chemistry and bodily response, misinterpret the signs as abnormal. Unnecessary anxiety may result over a sense of performance failure.

When people encounter a sudden decrease in sexual interest or capacity, typically the cause is not the normal tides of life but other problems. Such dysfunctions involve a lack of desire for or pleasure from sexual activity; an inability to experience or control orgasm; or a physiological obstacle that inhibits sexual arousal or interaction. Again, sexual problems, in both men and women, are often accompanied by a sense of distress or disappointment at the inability to participate in the sexual relationship.

Too often in older people a sexual problem is overlooked or untreated. The patient does not report the problem to the doctor out of embarrassment, or the physician fails to address the issue even after learning of it. Some doctors still take the attitude that medicine has maintained for generations, namely that sexual dysfunction is to be expected, a predictable and problematic consequence of aging, disease, or treatment.

ERECTILE DYSFUNCTION. Formerly known by the misleading term "impotence," erectile dysfunction describes a man's inability to obtain an erection sufficient to have sexual intercourse. It is a commonplace problem (perhaps thirty million American men, most of them over fifty) have chronic erection difficulties. But it is also estimated that as many as 90 percent of cases of erectile dysfunction can be improved or entirely resolved with proper diagnosis and treatment.

Sometimes the problem isn't a physical problem; if the erectile dysfunction occurs suddenly and its course is unpredictable, the cause is likely to be psychological. The loss of a spouse or intense emotional stress are common explanations. On the other hand, if the erectile failure has developed slowly over a period of months, the odds are that the cause is a physical illness. Underlying causes can be diabetes, hypertension, multiple sclerosis, traumatic injury, or one (or more) of a number of medications, including certain tranquilizers, antidepressants, and antihypertensives in the beta-blocker family. Alcohol and nicotine can also play a role.

Treatment. First consult your physician. A physical exam, an evaluation of your history, and an assessment of your alcohol and medication use may provide clues. Erectile dysfunction can also be evaluated by sleep studies, during which a portable home monitor records your erections during sleep.

In recent years, a number of prescription drugs have proven highly effective and popular in treating male erectile dysfunction and impotence. Although originally tested as a treatment for hypertension and angina, sildenafil citrate (Viagra) was found to produce penile erections. Approved by the FDA as a treatment for erectile dysfunction in 1998, sildenafil and its various competitors, vardenafil (Levitra), and tadalafil (Cialis), have been used by tens of millions of men to treat erectile dysfunction. All these drugs (called phosphodiesterase type 5 inhibitors, or PDE5s, for short) require a doctor's prescription. These drugs may pose a risk for people with cardiovascular disease and cause certain side effects, including headaches, dizziness, and, rarely, hearing loss. They have proven effective for roughly two-thirds of those who have taken them, including men with diabetes, multiple sclerosis, heart disease, and a wide range of other conditions. Talk to your physician.

The immense profitability of the PDE5s has led drug pharmaceutical companies to pursue wide-ranging research to identify drugs to treat women's sexual dysfunctions, too. One line of investigation involves a testosterone patch that, though not yet approved for general use, may help increase sexual desire and satisfaction. (Testosterone, the primary male hormone, appears to influence sexual desire in both men and women, though women typically have much smaller amounts in their bodies.)

Psychotherapy. Because nearly all sexual problems and intimacy issues involve the emotions, talking to a professional about the problem can be an effective part of treatment. A psychotherapist, sex therapist, marriage counselor, or another professional may provide an opportunity to explore, understand, and address past issues as well as current concerns.

Aging involves many changes that can impact one's sexuality. The shift in orientation from career and success that comes with retirement may require a new understanding of relationships. When facing physical deterioration and decline, you may need to reach a new understanding of changing circumstances. Larger life issues—considering your own mortality, life course events, past experiences, mourning the loss of a friend or loved one—can inform and affect your sexuality and need for intimacy. Impor-

PRESCRIPTION II

YOUR THREE STRATEGIES TO VITAL INTERPERSONAL CONNECTIONS

Central to this chapter is a three-step prescription; it requires a commitment of time and concentration. The promise is a more vital life. To review:

Strategy Four: Maintaining Friendships

What have you done to nurture your caring connections? To review the ways you can enhance your friendly behaviors, see page 63.

Strategy Five: Making New Friends

Have you found ways of making new acquaintances who, over time, may become valued friends? For suggestions, see page 67.

Strategy Six: Maintaining Sexual Communication

Our sexuality evolves over the years; have you found a means of communicating about the changes with your partner? For possible ways, see page 76.

Finding means of connecting in vital ways to friends and family can enhance healthy aging.

tant social relationships can be harmed by sexual problems, too. Seeking help can often resolve the problem.

Friendship, Sex, and Sharing

Loyalty, passion, romance, and simple friendship require two people; a pair of independent people brought together in a mutual satisfying way affirms our humanity. The life of the individual is enhanced by such connections.

Sexuality is an intimate form of human expression. Sex informs and enriches our lives. It can make us feel alive. We can experience and share the unique pleasures that sexuality brings to human existence. It can affirm our identities. By sharing sex with a partner, you can affirm that despite the decades, passion remains.

The forms of friendship are varied. Closeness to others—the shared confidence of friends, the mutual intimacy of lovers—allows us to continue to grow and learn about ourselves. Friendship is both enduring and transient; the focus of relationships is simultaneously on a shared past and an expected future.

PRESCRIPTION III

SEEK ESSENTIAL SLEEP

❖

SLEEP IS FUNDAMENTAL TO GOOD HEALTH, GOOD SPIRITS, AND longevity. To put it another way, quality of sleep is inextricably linked to quality of life. It is not a luxury for the lazy; sleep is essential for everyone.

Poor sleeping habits have been linked to the genesis of disease. To cite just one recent example, a study published in 2007 drew upon the life histories of some ten thousand British civil servants in midlife over a period of more than dozen years. The investigators concluded on the basis of their data that too little sleep—or, interestingly, too *much* sleep—put participants at a greater risk of death from cardiovascular disease.

Researchers have repeatedly found how important a good night's sleep is. Several years ago, I convened an interdisciplinary workshop at the International Longevity Center to look at the critical topic of sleep. A dozen professionals gathered to consider what we know about sleep and aging—

and what we need to know, to study, and to examine further. Much of what follows represents the consensus of our discussions.

Sleep enables the body to do repair work, as muscle cells and brain neurons are regenerated while we sleep. The sleeping brain consolidates emotional and social experiences, forms new synaptic connections, and encodes and sorts memories. Unfortunately, after age sixty-five more than half of us experience sleep problems, which can compromise some of these essential functions.

While a good night's rest is restorative and protective, sleep deprivation negatively affects the memory and, with too little rest, our mental and physical skills can rapidly deteriorate. Too little sleep—or, to use the catchall term for sleeping difficulties, *insomnia*—may make one feel, quite simply, old and tired. As someone who has suffered from periods of insomnia all his life, I speak from experience. Too little sleep probably produces a loss of immune function, too, since researchers have found that people who stay awake seventy-two consecutive hours experience a significant drop in white blood cell action and reproduction. Insufficient sleep has been linked to high blood pressure, and sleep deprivation has been shown to produce a prediabetic state in some individuals.

While lots of aging people have quite normal sleep patterns, others find that a good night's sleep becomes more elusive. We envy the teenagers who can sleep until noon; they do not even appreciate how delicious is the pleasure of deep, undisturbed sleep. We may find our internal alarm clocks awaken us even on days when we do not have to rise at a work-a-day hour.

Yet when it comes to sleep among older people, researchers have also produced reassuring findings. The old dogma that poor sleep is an inevitable part of aging is simply not true: Age in itself is not a predictor of insomnia and, when insomnia occurs, it is precipitated by other factors, many of which can be changed or compensated for. You can take steps to maintain or restore the homeostatic process of sleep by enabling the body's internal clock to shift appropriately from waking to sleeping, and there are common causes, among them obesity, alcohol consumption, nasal conges-tion, excessive snoring, medications, nicotine, and overeating, which can be treated.

In short, many things can produce sleeplessness, but aging in itself prob-ably isn't one of them. And if you have trouble sleeping, a range of strategies you will find in the pages to come can be employed to help reestablish healthy sleep patterns and enhance your life during the three-decade dividend.

The Mechanism of Sleep

One way to understand how the sleep cycle works is to observe it when it malfunctions. Take the case of Alisa Laughlin, a woman in her late middle years who, at first, did not even know she had a sleeping problem. Certainly she knew she was tired during the day; in fact, over a period of months her drowsiness began to interfere with her ability to keep up with the myriad details so critical to operating her travel agency. When she lost one of her most reliable customers—he got to San Francisco and found she had failed to make him a hotel reservation—she went to her doctor.

She complained that she was tired all the time, but it was an offhand comment that proved to be the essential clue for her physician. She re-ported that she woke up in the night. "I do not even know how many times!" she said, exasperated. Her physician arranged for her to undergo a sleep study, and she spent a night at the sleep laboratory at her local hospi-tal. She slept in a private room while a technician in a nearby monitoring area kept close watch on her sleeping activity. What he observed confirmed her doctor's diagnosis. She did indeed "awaken" often; that is, she stopped breathing, snorted loudly, stirred but did not truly wake up, and then went back to sleep, only to go through the process again and again, dozens of time per hour.

"Sleep apnea," her doctor told Alisa. He also told her she was one of millions of Americans with the disorder. Fortunately, he could offer her a solution, a specially designed oxygen mask that enabled her to breathe consistently through the night.

Plain and simple, she says, "It has changed my life."

Strategy Seven: Set Yourself Up for Sleep

The task is to take appropriate precautions to be sure you are not sabotaging your sleep. Many people develop habits over time that can interfere with a good night's sleep. You may be among them.

THE ASSIGNMENT. My prescription is as follows:

1. Read the following advisories and note two new behaviors you can adopt to improve your sleep.
2. Identify two bad habits you have that you can change.

TIPS FOR SLEEPING WELL. These advisories may help you sleep better:

- *Keep yourself busy.* Too little to do during the day—not enough exercise, too much time in bed, too many naps, insufficient mental activity—may be a factor in impaired sleep.
- *Limit caffeine consumption.* Avoid caffeinated beverages in the afternoon and evening or altogether; in sensitive individuals, even a small amount of caffeine in the morning can produce wakefulness at night.
- *Be certain your medications are not keeping you up.* Many medications act as stimulants, so check to be sure that wakefulness, disturbed sleep, insomnia, or another sleeping problem is not a result of your medication(s). If you think any of the prescription or over-the-

counter medications you are taking might be interfering with your sleep, discuss alternative therapies with your physician.

- *Avoid alcohol.* Beer, wine, and spirit consumption disrupts sleep, especially when taken to excess (see *Alcohol: Tonic or Toxin?* on page 193).
- *Limit liquid intake in the evening.* A major reason for sleep interruption in the night is the need to urinate, so moderate your consumption of liquids late in the day.
- *Exercise earlier.* Timing can be important: Late afternoon exercise is probably best, but make sure it's at least three hours before bedtime.
- *Take a nap a day to sleep the night away.* A short nap—no more than twenty to thirty minutes—can be good for you.
- *. . . But beware excess napping.* A long nap or more than one short one per day can ruin a good night's sleep. Napping late in the day—say, after three o'clock—can also interfere with your night's sleep.
- *Go for a walk.* Walking is good exercise; if conditions permit, walking outdoors will also increase your exposure to light and help to cue the brain's wake-sleep cycle.
- *Do not smoke.* Nicotine is a stimulant and can even cause nightmares.
- *Avoid eating heavy meals in the evening.* Too much food too close to bedtime can lead to difficulty sleeping.
- *. . . But do not go to bed hungry.* Feeling hungry can also interfere with your ability to sleep. Try eating a light snack in the hours before bedtime.
- *Keep a regular schedule.* Consistency in the time of retiring and rising can help entrain your body; too much variation can confuse the works.

- *Establish a bedtime routine.* Avoid activities that make you anxious in the hours before bedtime; instead, plan a routine that relaxes you.
- *Find some relaxation strategies.* Hot baths, long walks, calming music or natural sounds, stretching regimes like yoga, and deep breathing have been found to help.
- *When sleeplessness sets in, do not fight it.* If you still feel wakeful after fifteen minutes of trying to settle down, take a break from sleeplessness. If you awaken in the night, experience restlessness, and cannot go back to sleep, accept your body's verdict. Read for a time; write in a journal; listen to an all-night classical radio station. When you feel tired again, go back to bed . . . and to sleep.

A Good Night's Sleep

For the average adult, seven to eight hours of sleep per night is desirable. Whatever their ages, most Americans do not sleep enough, as the average tends to be more like six and a half hours a night. (Note, however, that some individuals do require less, and remain healthy and function well on as few as three to fours hours of sleep per night; they are the exceptions.)

So how much sleep is enough for you? I take a commonsense approach to answering the question: A good night's sleep is one that leaves you feeling well rested and able to function at your best throughout the day. It does not have to be any more complicated than that.

The normal sleep-wake cycle follows a daily pattern established by the body's internal clock. The so-called *circadian rhythms* (from the Latin words *circa* and *dies*, meaning "about the day") are actually a pattern of daily changes in the body's workings. These include variations in body temperature, which begins to rise very early in the morning before we awaken and falls at night. The SCN, or suprachiasmatic nuclei, in the brain's hypothalamus issues instructions to the pineal gland, a pea-sized structure tucked between the brain's hemispheres. As the darkness of the day settles in, the gland secretes melatonin, the hormone that helps initiate the resting process. Melatonin sends the signal that it is time to sleep; during the day, levels of melatonin in the body are so low as to be almost undetectable. New findings reported in 2009 from the NIH suggest that the pineal gland actually plays an important role in a surprising variety of body functions, interacting with genes that control body activities as diverse as cholesterol production and inflammation.

Sleep is not a constant state. Using the electroencephalograph (EEG), an instrument that records brain activity using electrodes attached to the scalp, researchers have found that, in the course of a normal night's rest, a sleeper experiences a series of sleep stages, each of which is identifiable in brain wave studies by its characteristic patterns. Stage 1 is the passage to sleep; sleepers awakened during Stage 1 are often convinced they have not been sleeping. During Stage 2 your breathing becomes regular, your body temperature drops, and your heart rate decreases. Roughly half of a night's sleep is spent in Stage 2.

Stages 3 and 4 are called deep sleep. These are times during which bones and muscles are built and tissues regenerated, and your breathing and brain activity slows still further. Blood pressure drops to its lowest levels. When awakened from Stage 4, the sleeper tends to think more slowly than usual and to feel groggy for thirty minutes or so.

The fifth stage of sleep is quite different from the others. It was first identified (and named) more than a half-century ago, when sleep researchers observed that at intervals the eyes of a sleeper seemed to flutter beneath his closed lids. Further investigation found that so-called rapid eye movement sleep (REM sleep) was characterized by increases in cerebral activity, heart rate, respiration, blood pressure, and blood flow to the brain. Periods of REM sleep usually last between five and twenty minutes. Even more intriguing, researchers found by awakening sleepers that most dreaming occurs during REM sleep. The brain waves during REM more nearly resemble those of wakefulness, and the body is effectively immobilized, which seems to be the brain's way of preventing us from acting out our dreams.

A night's sleep consists of alternating periods of Non-REM, or NREM, sleep (as Stages 1 through 4 are classified) and REM sleep. The sleeper descends first through Stages 1 to 4, then reverses the sequence, culminating with a period of REM sleep. The combined cycle typically lasts about one and a half to two hours, and a normal night's sleep consists of three to six such NREM-REM cycles.

The precise functions of sleep remain uncertain, although theories abound. REM sleep probably is a time when distant but linked memories are processed and stored. Studies have found that people deprived of REM sleep have a lesser ability to retain patterns learned the previous day (the loss of NREM sleep has no such effect). REM sleep may also be a time when the brain, like an overloaded computer, reorganizes itself. Another working theory has it that the cortex, the complex outer layer of the brain where we do our thinking, needs complete rest from time to time, and sleep provides it. Dreams probably also play a role in managing stress, regulating mood, and exercising the imagination.

In contrast, Stage 4 is thought to be restorative, a time when our body conserves energy, the nervous system recuperates, and the brain replenishes itself biochemically. In young people, sleep is a busy time for growth and development. Perhaps the body as a whole also requires a time of energy conservation.

Despite the ongoing research into the functions of sleep, the question as to why we spend a third of our lives immobile and largely unconscious remains an assemblage of intriguing guesswork. But we do know that even short-term interruptions of the circadian rhythms, such as those that occur with the time-zone shifts of jet lag, can produce insomnia, fatigue, and disorientation. When the normal sleep-wake cycle is disrupted for a sustained period for any reason, you may experience the sensation of sleepiness or even tend to fall asleep at odd times, as your brain tries to compensate for sleep deprivation. It is your body's way of encouraging you to sleep longer and more deeply.

THE AGING SLEEPER. In healthy older people, sleep does not change radically with the passing years. Certainly there are a number of subtle alterations to be observed, as sleep tends to be lighter, with less Stage 4 or deep sleep. Brief awakenings (typically three to ten seconds) are more common, and a night's sleep tends to shorten by perhaps half an hour. The time required to fall asleep (a period called "sleep latency") grows a bit longer; in the young, sleep may seem to come immediately, while in aging people ten minutes or more may be required to drift off. While a twenty-something will likely be sleeping 95 percent of the night, aging people snooze a bit less, perhaps for 85 percent of the sleep period.

These are incremental changes and healthy people adapt well, finding that the effects are not such that they complain of disturbed sleep or insomnia. Researchers have also found that the mature sleep patterns of a sixty-year-old are unlikely to change very much over the decades that follow unless there is a significant alteration of health status.

In my clinical practice, I have observed that serious sleep disorders are most often associated with growing medical burdens. Chronic pain can produce wakefulness; in fact, studies have found that pain leads not only to sleep deprivation but a cycle in which the loss of sleep actually increases the sen-

LONGEVITY AWARENESS CHECK

Ask yourself these questions:

Q: Did you get between seven and eight hours of relatively uninterrupted sleep last night?

Q: Do you have to rely on a prescription sleeping remedy to help you sleep?

Q: Does your spouse or partner complain that you snore long and loudly?

Q: Have your sleeping habits changed (that is, you're getting less sleep) significantly in the last five years?

Q: Would you trade almost anything for a good night's sleep?

The vital life involves a pattern of regular and sustained sleep to keep the mind and body healthy and at full function.

sation of pain, which in turn engenders sleeplessness. Arthritis, the lung ailment chronic obstructive pulmonary disorder (COPD), and coronary heart disease are common causes of insomnia. Just as one consequence of poor health all too often is disordered sleep, the reverse is also true; if a medical illness gets resolved, chances are the sleep problem will be, too.

sleeping potions—good news and bad

Resorting to a sleeping draught has a long and honorable tradition that extends back to Shakespeare and before. But as the story of Juliet Capulet suggests, the effects can be unpredictable. I don't recommend sleep medications except for occasional use or in the very short term. If, however, you opt for a sleep med, do the following:

- *Talk it over with the doctor.* Before using sleeping medications of any sort, consult your physician. Aging people with heart disease, hypertension, depression, and other disorders may be discouraged from using hypnotics or sedatives; there may also be a risk of drug interactions with other medications you are taking.
- *Abstain from alcohol.* Mixing drink and sleeping drugs is dangerous.
- *Take it at bedtime.* Timing is important: A sleeping medication taken too early can lead to premature sleepiness, impaired judgment, and loss of coordination.
- *Think short-term.* Sleeping pills may help you catch up on some lost sleep, but these medications do not treat the underlying causes and therefore should not be regarded as the solution to a chronic problem. Seek other solutions and strategies.
- *Report side effects.* If you experience any side effects—which can range from next-day drowsiness to weight gain—consult your physician. Note that over-the-counter sleeps aids can have side effects, too.
- *Discuss discontinuance.* When you decide to stop taking a sleeping medication, talk to your doctor. When discontinued after a sustained period of use, certain sleeping pills can produce rebound insomnia. A gradual decrease in dosage may be the wisest course.

Sleep Problems

Almost everyone experiences occasional sleeping difficulties, ranging from the college student stressed by tomorrow's test to the worried parent wondering at her child's temper tantrums. An estimated one in three adults suffers regularly from sleeplessness, and with the passing years such problems become more common. According to some studies, at least one in two older adults complains of significant sleep disruption. As we grow older, the body seems less able to compensate for sleep loss.

In spite of the fact that chronic sleep problems occur more often among older adults, poor sleep is not a natural—and therefore not a guaranteed—part of the aging process. Current research suggests that sleep after age sixty does not change much. But life can, and alterations in your life and health changes can precipitate sleep problems. The mourning that follows the death of someone close, for example, or the change of life brought on by your (or your partner's) retirement can affect sleep. A decrease in patterns of physical activity can lead to sleeplessness, too; perhaps surprisingly, a reduction in exposure to sunlight can also be a factor. Sleeplessness can also piggyback on itself: Disturbed sleep may redouble as a result of bodily changes in hormone levels or metabolism that are themselves the result of too little sleep.

When they occur, sleep problems should not be merely accepted as inevitable. If a good night's sleep is not a guaranteed right, it is at least an achievable goal for most people given good habits, healthy sleep strategies, and other widely available treatment approaches.

Sleep problems in older people tend to be associated with a range of ailments that are common to the age group, including diabetes, hypertension, depression, lung disease, and heart disease, each of which can affect an individual's sleep patterns. Pain of most any sort can affect sleep, and some medications result in disordered sleep, too. So let's look at some of the sleep problems that are common to the aging years.

INSOMNIA. The most common sleep complaint at any age is insomnia, the inability to sleep during the usual resting hours. Insomnia may be characterized by a difficulty in falling asleep, wakefulness after an initial period of sleep, or both. Half of all adult Americans report experiences with insomnia, and perhaps one in five of those experience insomnia significant enough that they find their waking activities impaired. They often report such varied symptoms as an inability to concentrate, slowed reaction time, memory difficulties, low spirits, generalized fatigue and sleepiness, excessive yawning, and difficulty in carrying out daily tasks. In older people, the risk of falling also increases with lost sleep.

Insomnia may be a short-term problem or a chronic condition. Acute insomnia may be caused by such life factors as bereavement or the adjustment to medical difficulties. Typically the problem is of short duration, and it generally improves without intervention or through the short-term use of sleeping pills called hypnotics (see *Medications*, page 100).

Chronic insomnia can result in reduced quality of life. Most insomnia is the result of something else, such as pain or discomfort from a medical condition or a behavior such as substance abuse, including alcohol consumption, or the use of certain prescription medications, among them such widely prescribed drugs as beta-blockers, bronchodilators, calcium-channel blockers, corticosteroids, decongestants, and thyroid hormones. Other potential causes of insomnia are depression, narcolepsy and other breathing-related sleep disorders, headaches, arthritis, or asthma.

SLEEP-DISORDERED BREATHING. Living with a snorer can be irritating; being one means facing a number of risks, ranging from the relatively minor to the potentially life threatening. Snoring can be a warning sign, an indicator of a serious health problem. A long-term study of nurses linked snoring with an increased risk of cardiovascular disease in women, independent of age, smoking, overweight, and other risk factors.

One impact of snoring is the restriction of oxygen reaching the bloodstream; this lack of oxygen causes the sleeper to wake up. A repeated pattern of oxygen deficiency in the blood (called hypoxemia) and abrupt arousals can also lead to increases in blood pressure. More men than women tend to experience sleep-disordered breathing. According to one study, roughly one in ten women and one in four men experience five or more breathing pauses and awakenings ("respiratory events") per night.

Snoring may seem harmless, but it should not be regarded as benign. While occasional snoring is at the milder end of the spectrum of sleep-disordered breathing, it tends to be progressive.

SLEEP APNEA. When the number of respiratory events rises to fifteen or more per hour, the clinical diagnosis of sleep apnea is applied. Some individuals with sleep apnea stop breathing hundreds of times per night, either because the soft tissues in the rear of the throat collapse and block the airway (obstructive sleep apnea, or OSA) or because the brain fails to signal the muscles to breathe (central sleep apnea, or CSA). Many with sleep apnea have a mix of both OSA and CSA.

The result of such nighttime arousals is fragmented sleep that, in turn, impairs attention, short-term memory, perceptual learning, and the acquisition of long-term memory, and may also lead to impotence and weight gain. Several studies have found that people who suffer from sleep apnea have high rates of automobile accidents. People with sleep apnea typically have no recollection of their nighttime awakenings in the morning.

The problem is common: According the National Institutes of Health estimates, perhaps twelve million Americans suffer from sleep apnea, many of them undiagnosed.

Risk factors associated with sleep apnea include obesity, alcohol consumption, smoking, nasal congestion, and, in menopausal women, estrogen depletion.

Treatment. Lifestyle changes can be effective in treating sleep-disordered breathing and, in some cases, sleep apnea. In overweight individuals, weight loss often relieves the symptoms, and can be achieved through a combination of a healthy diet and regular exercise. Avoiding alcohol or discontinuing certain medications (such as sedatives) that relax the central nervous system may also prove helpful. If you are a smoker, a diagnosis of sleep-disordered breathing or sleep apnea is a very good reason to quit.

Some people with sleep apnea find relief when they employ special pillows or devices that prevent them from sleeping on their backs. Oral appliances are also available to help keep the airway open during sleeping. If such conservative therapies prove inadequate, your physician may recommend the use of nasal continuous positive air-pressure (CPAP). This therapy provides a continuous flow of oxygen through a face mask attached via a tube to a machine that blows pressurized air. Sometimes surgery is also recommended to remove tissues and clear the airway.

If you or another member of your household appears to have sleep apnea, consult a doctor.

RESTLESS LEG SYNDROME. The name quite neatly describes the discomfort: It occurs when a tingling, aching, itching, or burning sensation in the legs is accompanied by an irresistible urge to move them when sitting or lying down. The unpleasant feeling is sometimes described as a sensation like that of insects crawling inside the leg. The cause is often unknown, although RLS seems to run in families and can even start in childhood. It may also accompany other conditions, including anemia and pregnancy in younger women, rheumatoid arthritis, and Parkinson's disease. It can also be a side effect of certain medications.

Treatment. As with many sleep disorders, the symptoms of RLS may be relieved by moderate exercise during the day and relaxation techniques prior to sleeping. If the onset is abrupt, a medication may have been the cause, so your physician may recommend avoiding certain drugs. Some antitremor and anticonvulsant medications can be helpful in severe and chronic cases.

Strategy Eight: Set the Scene for Sleep

The goal is to sleep better or longer. There may be very simple lifestyle steps you can take to enhance your night's rest.

THE ASSIGNMENT. Look to make your daily life more sleep-friendly.

1. Try to think about bedtime as a process: Sleeping, resting, and napping are all about letting go. Falling asleep requires that you disengage from your waking life and slide into a restful unconsciousness.
2. Incorporate into your bedtime ritual some of the approaches listed below.

SLEEP, PERCHANCE TO DREAM. Here are some sleepy-time ideas:

- *Slow your pace.* In the hours before bedtime, consciously slow the rhythm of the day to help you settle into the sleep phase. Your body temperature naturally begins to drop in the evening, a metabolic sign that the time for rest is coming.
- *Send the right signal to your mind and body.* The bedroom should feel comfortable (cool, perhaps, but not cold). Loud noises, either sustained or intermittent, do not help you relax, so do what you need to do to assure peace and quiet during sleeping hours. Sound insulation, bedroom relocation, or shifting household activities may help.
- *Make going to bed a ritual.* Do it at a consistent time. Have a hot bath ninety minutes before bedtime; plan a thirty-minute period of relaxation before retiring.
- *Recognize the messenger.* Darkness is a sign-giver that your brain recognizes as a prompt to shift into sleep mode; your natural circadian rhythms are adapted to the cues of the sun. Use such sign-givers to your advantage: Curtains, for example, can shield you from bright lights at night and early-morning sunlight.
- *Consider your comfort.* How comfortable is your mattress? If yours feels like the princess's pea has grown into a pumpkin, buy a new

one. Many affordable models are available. Or you may choose to splurge—the premium mattress today would be almost unrecognizable to past generations, with its quilted top, open-cell foams that "remember" your imprint, increase airflow, and other technical advancements. A more comfortable mattress just might translate into a better night's sleep.

- *Adopt strategies to reduce your anxiety level.* A notebook next to the bed can relieve you of your *Oops, I forgot* thoughts; write down the forgotten task and forget about it until tomorrow.

- *Keep the excitement level low.* Think of the bed as a place for sleep and sex only; if your mind associates the bed with exciting ball games on TV or up-tempo activities, sleep may be harder to come by.

- *Let it happen.* Just as you cool down after a workout, let the intensity of the day slip away. For some people, bedtime reading is more effective than a sedative. Choose carefully: Novels full of conflict or violence, tracts that raise your political ire, or news stories that leave you worrying about the state of the world will not help you sleep.

Ensuring a Good Night's Sleep

There are some eighty known sleep problems and disorders, ranging from the commonplace to the obscure. For minor or occasional sleep problems, the practical strategies in this chapter may help you resolve the problem yourself.

On the other hand, your sleep problem may rise to the level of a medical problem, one that you should discuss with your physician. According to the National Sleep Foundation, one or more of the following warning signs argue for consulting the doctor:

- If you snore loudly.
- If you or others have observed that you stop breathing or gasp for breath during sleep.
- If you feel sleepy or doze off while watching TV, reading, driving, or performing other daily activities.
- If you have difficulty sleeping three nights a week or more (e.g., trouble falling asleep, awakening frequently during the night, waking too early, inability to get back to sleep, or not feeling refreshed upon rising).
- If you experience unpleasant, tingling, creeping feelings or nervousness in your legs when trying to sleep.
- If you experience regular sleep interruptions like nighttime heartburn, bad dreams, or pain.

Studies have found that many people do not report sleep problems to their physicians, but keep in mind, once again, that sleep problems are not a given in the aging years. Make your doctor a partner in your care and share your sleep issues with him or her, along with your other aches, complaints, and concerns.

There are other factors you should be aware of.

WEIGHT CONTROL. The most important risk factor for sleep-disordered breathing is overweight. Studies have shown that even modest weight loss can have a positive effect, so follow up on that resolution to shed a few pounds. If you are not sure whether you are overweight, consult the *Body Mass Index*, page 141. See also *Prescription VII: Eat Your Way to Health*, page 179, for sound nutritional strategies.

A NAP A DAY? I have already mentioned that a nap can be helpful. That said, too much napping during the day is likely to worsen nocturnal sleepless-ness. On the other hand, there is evidence that a brief afternoon nap can help relieve daytime sleepiness and improve evening alertness.

You must use your good sense: You know whether your mind and body crave sleep at times other than the usual sleeping hours. And you need not feel guilty giving in: Taking a regular nap does not imply indolence; the reward for a nap can be better concentration and a lift in attitude.

Again, keep your nap short: twenty to thirty minutes in a darkened room, at the same time each day, is ideal. Another incentive may be the finding, published in 2007, of a large Greek study involving men between ages twenty and eighty. The investigators found that those who napped about thirty minutes a day were 30 percent less likely to develop heart disease. Call it an added potential bonus.

COGNITIVE BEHAVIOR THERAPY. A branch of psychotherapy called cognitive therapy seeks to enable the patient to identify thoughts, assumptions, and behaviors that are not helpful and to change them. The cognitive behavioral therapist treating sleeping problems will seek to help you associate the bedroom with sleep; to train you to relax; and to employ sleep restriction therapy, in which you devise and adopt a new sleeping schedule to minimize wakefulness and maximize sleep during the sleeping hours. If you feel as if your sleep regimen is disordered, cognitive therapy may prove useful.

MEDICATIONS. An old truism has it that magic answers in life are rare; that rule applies to sleeping pills, too. While they certainly help some people (in 2008, American consumers spent more than four billion dollars on sleeping medications), the benefits, according to most studies, could hardly be described as remarkable.

The results of one study published in 2006 are illuminating. On the one hand, the researchers found that participants who used the new generation of sleeping pills fell asleep more quickly and slept longer those who took placebos. Yet this NIH-funded study also found that the subjects gained an average of *less than twelve minutes of sleep* per night while drifting off to sleep some thirteen minutes faster. Such outcomes are undoubtedly welcome to those with insomnia, but these drugs are no panacea. Nevertheless, the stock response of many physicians is to prescribe sleeping pills; roughly half of all patients who complain to their doctors of insomnia are treated with one or another of the hypnotics, a class of drugs used to induce sleep.

The medications marketed to help you sleep fall into basic two categories. The hypnotics are the class of drugs used to induce sleep. These include the generic zaleplon (sold under the brand name Sonata) and zolpidem (Ambien). A second class of prescription medication, the hypnotic-sedatives, are prescribed to help you stay asleep. Widely used hypnotic-sedatives include eszopiclone (Lunesta), temazepam (Restoril), and zolpidem (Ambien CR). Another drug, ramelteon (Rozerem), works by enhancing the receptivity of the brain to melatonin. These medications are usually prescribed only as short-term treatments, typically for less than two weeks.

Cost can be a factor: Three and four dollars per pill is the going rate for some of the newer drugs, meaning a two-week regimen prices out in the fifty-dollar range.

Side effects. Some individuals who take sleeping medications experience unwanted side effects. Headache, dizziness, and prolonged drowsiness can occur. Some users report episodes of sleep-driving and sleep-eating in the night. Evidence also suggests that in older adults, the use of sleeping medications increases the risk of falls and injury.

No sleeping medications should be mixed with alcohol. The addition of alcohol to the bloodstream can multiply the sedative effects, potentially leading to confusion, dizziness, and fainting or, in the case of overdose, even death. Sleep disturbances can worsen when, after a period of use, a drug is discontinued, as rebound insomnia and nightmares may occur.

OTHER THERAPIES. If your body's circadian rhythms are clearly out of phase, your physician may recommend *bright light therapy*, in which you spend prescribed periods every day exposed to intense light. The source may be a specially designed light box, desk lamp, or a light visor, which will resynchronize your sleep patterns.

YOUR TWO STRATEGIES TO A BETTER NIGHT'S SLEEP

The prescription of this chapter is to sleep better. Essential to accomplishing that is to allow it to happen by avoiding certain behaviors and by setting the right circumstances. The promise of better sleep is a strong sense of vitality during your waking day.

Strategy Seven: Set Yourself Up for Sleep

Many activities we pursue doing the day can, by their nature or timing, interfere with our rest. Changing certain patterns or habits can enable you to sleep better. To review some options, see page 86.

Strategy Eight: Set the Scene for Sleep

Make your bedroom a haven from the excitement of the world; it should be your escape. For suggestions, see page 96.

Sleep can add clarity, a feeling of well-being, and even confidence to your day.

PRESCRIPTION IV

SET STRESS
ASIDE

❖

IF YOU ARE FEELING STRESSED OUT, YOU COULD BE MAKING yourself sick. Over time, too much stress can lead to sleep deprivation, overeating, substance abuse, and other health-damaging behaviors. The long-term consequences can be wear and tear on the body that, in turn, can play a role in the development of such conditions as obesity, type-2 diabetes, brain atrophy, heart disease, loss of sexual function, high blood pressure, stroke, loss of muscle and bone strength, suppression of the body's immune system, and depression.

The message? *Get your stress under control.*

If the threat of those diseases isn't enough incentive, consider the results of a 2008 study conducted at the University of Washington that demonstrated that stress affects cognition, too. Rats subjected to stressors (in this

Is your life too stressful?

Q: *Do you feel pressured all the time?*

Q: *Does the day seem like a rush to nowhere?*

Q: *Do you often feel preoccupied, worried, or that you are running behind?*

Q: *Are you easily distracted? Do you have trouble focusing on a task or concentrating when you read?*

Q: *Does it sometimes feel as if the weight of the universe rests on your shoulders?*

Q: *Do you feel the need to do everything yourself?*

Q: *Are you impatient with coworkers or irritable with friends and family?*

Q: *Does your work interfere with your family life?*

Q: *Would you describe your eating patterns as disordered? Do you race through meals, stuffing yourself, or starve yourself, either intentionally or out of inattention?*

Q: *Do you often experience physical discomforts such as a stiff neck, recurrent headache, sore back, or stomach pain?*

Q: *Is your mouth frequently dry and your palms sweaty? Do you find yourself unconsciously tapping your fingers and feet in impatience?*

Q: *Do you sleep poorly? Do you have difficulty finding time to exercise?*

Q: *Do you self-medicate with alcohol to relax? Have you a noticed a gradual increase in your alcohol consumption? Do you smoke?*

Q: *Do you feel as if you have little control over day-to-day events?*

Q: *Have you no means whereby you can truly relax on a regular basis?*

No single "yes" answer means you are stressed out and endangering your health, but if you answered more than a third of these questions in the affirmative, you can live a more vital life by lessening your stress.

case random electric shocks to their tails) were about 25 percent less likely to make correct decisions in seeking a water source. Tests in humans have found that too much stress can interfere with the brain's executive function, such as the decision-making process concerning food intake.

At the risk of oversimplifying, let's just say that stress can make you sick—and it can make you behave less intelligently. Thus, there are numerous reasons to reduce the stress in your life.

Understanding Stress

There are two types of stress. The first, *acute stress*, may save your life in an emergency, enabling you to react when confronted by an urgent situation. The human body responds with what is understood to be the "fight or flight response." Upon encountering a perceived danger, the nervous system stimulates an immediate rise in heart rate and blood pressure, which provides our muscles with needed oxygen. The immune system prepares to deal with infection or injury; the alerted brain becomes more vigilant; energy stores in the liver are mobilized; and growth and digestion are temporarily suspended. In short, *an acute stress reaction* prepares us for action.

The other kind of stress reaction, however, is not protective. This kind of stress reaction, called *chronic stress*, is a health hazard that can reduce the body's ability to maintain normal physiologic and cognitive function, undermining mental concentration and the ability to solve problems. The impact of such stress on various bodily systems can be large and, over time, even life-threatening. Sustained stress can compromise the health of your cardiovascular and gastrointestinal systems, and excess stress has been found to destroy brain cells and lessen the immune system's ability to fight infection and heal wounds. In animal trials, chronic stress has been linked to everything from digestive diseases to overweight and underweight, excessive alcohol consumption, anxiety disorders, loss of fur, skin disorders, and skin and ovarian cancers. In humans, chronic stress is linked to sleep problems, gastrointestinal complaints, and anxiety.

Stress illustrates something important about the human animal: Good and bad health often begin in the brain. It makes sense given the myriad ways in which the brain orchestrates the body's responses. Yet modern medicine is very much invested in trying to understand the machinery of the body from the neck down, looking at cells and molecules and genes. All of that is important, but often the approach fails to take into consideration the vital input of our lives, such as the social context, our life events, and our emotional responses.

To manage stress in our lives, we need to look at the way we react to our world. If we respond in a way that produces stress, we put our health at risk—and threaten our ability make the most of our added decades and even our longevity. The goal here is to help you find a healthy balance so you can respond to a sudden emergency but turn the stress response off again when it is no longer needed. That will help you maintain optimal physical and mental fitness.

mood music

Do kids get smarter just by listening to Mozart? Proponents of the so-called Mozart Effect think so. Perhaps, then, it is not surprising that many adults find that music has salubrious effects, too.

In one study a group of patients were given the opportunity to listen to music of their choice immediately before cataract surgery. Within five minutes, researchers found, the patients' blood pressure and heart rate, which had been elevated in anticipation of the procedure, returned to normal levels. A control group that had been offered no music to listen to experienced higher than normal blood pressure and heart rates during and after surgery.

A Japanese study found that music helped relieve back pain. There is also evidence of music's utility in treating depression. Music therapy is commonly used in helping cancer patients control pain and nausea. Some research suggests music reduces pain during dental procedures.

Ever noticed how long-lived classical conductors are? Even before the burst of longevity of recent years, men like Arturo Toscanini, Leopold Stokowski, Eugene Ormandy, and Arthur Fiedler guided their orchestras until well beyond retirement age (they lived to eighty-nine, ninety-five, eighty-five, and eighty-four years of age, respectively). Pianist Arthur Rubinstein still concertized at eighty-nine, even though his vision was so blurred he not only could not read music but he was unable to distinguish his fingers on the keyboard.

Much research remains to be done (there is strong disagreement among epidemiologists, for example, as to whether music is truly a causative factor in the longevity of conductors). But we do know that, if we allow it, stress can ride us like the cowboy on the bronco. If, on the other hand, we can throw it off, we can be healthier—and the therapeutic power of music in stress reduction may well be of help.

Find a way to enjoy the music you like in your everyday life. The options these days are widely varied, thanks to not only radios and CD players but the portable devices called MP3 players (for example, the Apple iPod). Music can be more than background; it can be grounding, relaxing, reassuring. It does not have to be classical music: For some people, country, pop, blues, folk, or a range of international styles makes life a little bit better.

How Stress Works

Let's examine the underlying mechanisms of stress.

Amid the immensely complex architecture of the brain is the limbic system, also called the paleomammalian brain. The limbic system performs multiple functions relating to our emotions, long-term memory, and behavior. One of its elements, the hippocampus, which is located deep in the brain, plays a key role in recording episodic memories of life's events. A nearby cluster of nerve cells, the amygdala, is the site for our experience of fear.

When we perceive a potential danger, the amygdala and hippocampus, together with the cerebral cortex, rapidly transmit the news to another area of the brain called the hypothalamus. In turn, this pea-size structure influences the heart, liver, immune system, and digestive organs through a fast, hardwired link of brain circuits called the *autonomic nervous system* (ANS). Hormonal messengers are dispatched—adrenaline, noradrenaline, cortisol, and acetylcholine—as well as brain messengers (neurotransmitters) like glutamate. Linked by neural circuitry to other brain regions such as the prefrontal cortex and the anterior cingulate cortex, this stress response system mobilizes us to deal with the challenge at hand. The involuntary bodily functions of the heart, certain glands (in particular salivary, stomach, and sweat glands), and the smooth muscles found in the internal organs, among other tissues, are affected, producing a constriction (shrinking) of the blood vessels and an increase in blood pressure. The heart accelerates while the stomach slows. The overall sensation you experience is hyperalertness: a readiness to flee or fight the bully in the schoolyard.

Once the challenge is removed or resolved, a calm follows that is akin to the silencing of a fire alarm. The branch of the autonomic nervous system called the *parasympathetic nervous system* alerts the body that the danger has passed. The production of the stress hormone cortisol by the hippocampus ceases. A memory of the stressful event is stored for future reference, and bodily processes return to normal function.

The response of the body to a challenge is protective and adaptive, but-wrepeated and prolonged chronic stress endangers health. Such chronic stress occurs when, in response to anxiety or the pressures of day-to-day events, the body remains on high alert. This is not merely the pressure of too much work or worry; chronic stress is a bodily state in which blood pressure remains high and cortisol levels elevated. The dynamic balance of the ANS is disrupted, and the resting heart rate remains elevated. Instead of rising during the day (when energy demand is higher) and decreasing at night, the heart beats in rigid regularity, failing to adapt to the cyclic demands of the day. This elevated heart rate has been associated with a wide range of health problems that extend across lines of gender and ethnicity. Once again, the risks include overweight, heart disease, hypertension, stroke, decreased immune system function, and depression.

Strategy Nine: Stress Reduction Through Exercise

Ever try to dribble an overinflated basketball? It is not difficult—the ball just bounces a bit higher and faster—but something is clearly wrong. Too much stress in your life makes you a bit like that basketball. You need to find an outlet to release tension.

THE ASSIGNMENT. The best stress-management strategies are twofold. On the one hand, you can employ your body to help your brain; on the other, your mind can reduce the stresses on your body. For this task I suggest you identify a means of exercise that can lessen the tension.

THE ACTIVITIES. A good workout will improve blood flow to the brain and will help you sleep. Exercise triggers the release of brain chemicals called endorphins, which can reduce anxiety levels, enhance our immune systems, and give us an overall feeling of well-being. In laboratory animals, fitness training has been found to decrease corticosteroid levels and enhance learning and memory. In humans, demonstrated benefits include treating mild to moderate depression, improving the ability to focus one's attention, and enhancing weight-loss regimes. Here are some guidelines.

- *Establish a basic schedule for regular exercise.* At a minimum, you should take three thirty-minute brisk walks a week.
- *More exercise is better.* Biking, jogging, swimming, taking aerobics classes, or other pastimes that involve vigorous, sustained motion are recommended.
- *Choose activities you enjoy doing.* If you do not, the best intentions in the world may soon fade to inaction.
- *Vary the regime.* Do it with a friend, integrate music, or otherwise find ways to make it enjoyable.
- *Be patient.* Being fit will also make you better able to deal with

life's challenges, whether they are day-to-day headaches or major events and illnesses. Chances are the good effects will be multifold, and you will feel better about yourself.

• For a range of exercise choices, see *Prescription VI: Live the Active Life,* page 138.

the relaxation response

Physicians today are more open to alternative therapies than they were a generation ago. Herbert Benson is one reason why.

As a young physician at Harvard Medical School, he conducted research into a pet hypothesis, namely that stress caused high blood pressure. Although he chose to pursue his investigations using squirrel monkeys in a laboratory in Cambridge, Dr. Benson was approached one day by a group of young people with their own theory of hypertension. They believed that by practicing Transcendental Meditation they reduced their blood pressure—and they wanted Dr. Benson to prove it in a clinical study. The notion seemed outlandish to some, but Benson launched what proved to be a landmark investigation into the effects of meditation.

He and his fellow researchers at Harvard and Beth Israel Hospital in Boston measured such bodily functions as metabolic rate, heartbeat, brain waves, and the rate of breathing, as well as blood pressure. The investigators took the readings before and after some of the subjects meditated for twenty minutes, while other participants in the study sat quietly. The findings rocked the medical world. By merely changing their thought patterns, the subjects demonstrably slowed their metabolism, brain activity, and breathing and heart rates.

Benson saw these changes as the opposite of the stress response, so he called it the *relaxation response.* Today Benson is widely recognized for his key role in exploring the so-called *mind-body connection;* his 1975 book *The Relaxation Response* was a hit and has helped millions learn how to relax.

TM technique is perhaps best learned in a workshop setting from a trained teacher. (Transcendental Meditation is a trademarked technique introduced by Maharishi Mahesh Yogi in 1958, based on an ancient Indian tradition.) But Benson's book and other practitioners can give you the basics. In essence, it involves a twenty-minute daily session in which you empty your mind, allowing it to "transcend" mental activity and reach a meditative state of relaxed alertness.

Strategy Ten: Change Your Thinking

Your thoughts play a crucial role in stress management. The brain is a key activator that, at both conscious and unconscious levels, disposes us to disease or tilts us toward health. The goal here is reduce stressors in your life for health and longevity.

THE ASSIGNMENT. I suggest you approach the challenge this way:

1. Think about a computer that's overwhelmed by too many complex tasks at once; it will crash.
2. Think about you under stress: Don't you feel as if your effectiveness has frozen up, too?
3. Find ways to reboot.

STRESS REDUCERS. Here are some different ways of thinking about our life.

* *Find quietude.* The human body is better able to counter or reduce the ravages of excess stress if you find the opportunity to escape the tension for a time. Exercise seems to be doubly effective in reducing stress when it is paired with such relaxation techniques as deep breathing, self-hypnosis, yoga, meditation (see *Taking a Deep Breath*, page 117, and *The Relaxation Response*, page 110). While training sessions, books, and other forms of guidance are available to help

you master specific techniques, you may already know how to find the calm you need. Once you identify it, take regular recourse to your personal place of escape.

- *Set limits.* Establish reasonable limits for work or other commitments; you cannot do it all. At the same time, allow for opportunities to pursue your own pleasures.
- *Reframe.* Look at your life through a different window. More than a few of the pressures you feel weighing on you are self-generated; rearranging your priorities may shift the burden. At times are you, metaphorically speaking, trying to move an object you know full well to be immovable? If you can't move the cliff face, perhaps you can find a boulder to roll? Try to step back from the noise and clutter and look at things from another angle. You can find elements to change or eliminate that are not necessary and that are not making your life better.
- *Do not insist on perfection.* Recognize that perfection is not always a reasonable or desirable goal either for you or those around you.
- *Keep a journal.* This may be news to you, but, according to several recent studies, putting your thoughts and feelings on paper is good for you. People with asthma and rheumatoid arthritis have been found to experience a lessening in symptoms when they write about their stress; another study found measurable decreases of stress hormones and fewer doctor visits among journalers. You may not be able to make your frustrations go away, but thinking them through and confiding them to a diary delivers benefits. You do not have to worry about getting a grade; there are no minimums or maximums. One common approach is putting pen to paper (or fingers to the keyboard) for fifteen minutes, say, three times a week. Get it off your chest. Today's problems, yesterday's complaints, long-ago torments, and tomorrow's worries are all fair game. You

may find opportunities for change, but even if you do not, understanding and accepting are in themselves healthful.

- *Skip the caffeine.* Less caffeine means less stimulation of your central nervous system. Keep in mind that caffeine is found in a number of products, including coffee, cola, chocolate, some teas, and many over-the-counter medications and dietary supplements. There are many people who swear by herbal teas such as ginseng and chamomile, but avoid teas that are billed as energizers, such as those containing ephedra.

- *Relinquish control.* As a control person, you know who you are.

- *Listen to music.* Loud, up-tempo music may not be the way to go, but that does not mean you have to settle for elevator music. You know what sort of music gives you a sense of ease. Let it take you for a ride—to someplace other than the "I must, I can't, I'm late, Oh, no!" world of the overstressed.

- *Get enough sleep.* For most people, that should mean seven to eight hours a night. (See *Prescription III: Seek Essential Sleep*, page 83.)

- *Reduce multitasking.* One of the great stress-inducers of modern times is the common compulsion to work, communicate (cell phone, text, e-mail), and manage your life all at once. You will be more efficient—and less stressed—if you segregate times and tasks.

- *Do not underestimate Mother Nature.* For many people, contact with the natural world has a restorative effect. Some report a new equilibrium after a walk in the woods, a few minutes spent observing birds at a feeder, or time spent watching a moonrise or a sunset. The natural world has a pace (the wind in the trees, the rolling of the waves, the soaring of a hawk in the thermals) that can remind us life does not have to be lived in a rush.

- *Keep flowers around.* A study at Kansas State University gave ninety women a five-minute typing assignment; researchers found that

those who worked with a bouquet of flowers at hand outper-
formed those with no flowers.

- *Reschedule.* Do not panic if your progress is slower than you wanted
  it to be. Stop, take a break to give you distance, then make a new
  plan and set a new end point.
- *Learn to negotiate.* Soften your hard stands—especially with
  yourself.
- *Pursue a favorite hobby.* Find the time to do what gives you pleasure
  and takes you out of the fast lane.
- *Change the tone.* Jumping out of bed to face the day is the right
  strategy for some; for others, though, a more gradual wake-up can
  set a less stressful tone. Instead of a jangling alarm, buy an inexpensive clock radio that will awaken you with music. Stretch before
  rising: Starting at your toes, flex all your muscles, working upward.
  You are looking to find an alignment, of sorts, that balances your
  mental, physical, and emotional life.
- *Simplify.* We do not crave chaos; on the contrary, most of us like a
  sense of control over our lives. Yet in our consumer society, objects accumulate around us: unanswered mail, yesterday's newspaper, gifts, collections, clothes, leftover bits of this and that. Begin
  by identifying everything on your kitchen counters, desk, entry
  hall, coffee table, and sideboard that you have not used in the last,
  say, six months. Sell, give, and trash at least half the items. Move
  the items you cannot part with to another place (a closet or a cup-
  board). Go through the ritual again every month. Friends will appreciate your kindness. You may get a few tax deductions. Your
  house will look less cluttered. And you will feel less stressed and
  more in control of your life.
- *Share your fears.* I promise you: You are not alone. Even in a time
  personal crisis—a death in the family, a lost job, divorce—there is
  someone out there to confide in. Tell a friend or relative of your

fears and feelings; if they seem too private to share with someone in your life, consult a psychotherapist. Many people find putting their worries down on paper (in a diary or a letter, for example) can help. Sometimes having written it down is enough; for some then tearing it up offers a sense of liberation. Do not just keep it in; find a way that works for you to let the feelings out.

- *Visualize.* You can use your mind, at no cost and with no equipment, to escape into your imagination. Relax, close your eyes, and think of a favorite spot: a sandy beach, a mountaintop, a remembered place from childhood where the warmth of happiness and security pervades. If you can explore the sounds, smells, and qualities of that recollection, you will find yourself *in the moment* in the best sense.

more laughter, please

Did you know that laughter reduces stress? Of course you did: Isn't it obvious how much better you feel after laughing? When a guffaw bursts forth, fifteen facial muscles are involved, along with the larynx, epiglottis, and lungs. A laugh is a noisy gasp and a physical act that releases sound, air, sometimes tears, and more.

Unlike most emotional reactions, laughter engages multiple sections of the brain, including the frontal lobe (where emotions are processed), the cerebral cortex (which helps process the information), and the occipital lobe (which controls the physical responses). Scientists in the pathology department at the Loma Linda School of Medicine demonstrated some of laughter's health-giving properties at a biological level some twenty years ago.

Ten men were chosen for the study. Five of them were shown a sixty-minute funny video; the other five were not. A series of blood samples revealed that the men who viewed the funny video had reduced levels of cortisol (an adrenal hormone associated with stress response), epinephrine (another hormone and a neurotransmitter), and growth hormone in their blood. The conclusion? "Mirthful laughter" (only a scientist would call a belly laugh "mirthful laughter") has "implications for the reversal of the neuroendocrine and classical stress hormone response." Translation? More laughter, less stress.

Is laughter really the best medicine? That's a big claim, but there is evidence, both scientific and anecdotal, that makes the case. In his classic book *Anatomy of an Illness*, the writer and magazine editor Norman Cousins described his experience in fighting a debilitating arthritic disease. In his experience, ten minutes of a Marx Brothers movie produced not merely mirth but also two hours of precious pain-free sleep. Other researchers have reported that laughter stimulates the release of endorphins in the brain.

Laughter seems to protect against heart disease, too, so find a way to put your funny bone to use. Maybe it is television or movies, books or comic strips, but a few mirthful chuckles will do you good.

Inverting the Equation

You cannot eliminate all stress from your life; stress is an unavoidable feature of our experience throughout the life course. Do not forget that some stress plays a key role in good health, enabling us to meet deadlines and to respond in an emergency, whether it is an event in the world or a personal medical trauma. But, as we've seen, stress also can set the stage for or trigger disease and disability.

There are many strategies cited earlier in this chapter, ranging from vigorous exercise to the motionlessness of meditation. You would be well advised to find a mix of techniques that suits you, and which you can integrate into your life. Be realistic and do not set your sights casually; think the process through so you will stay with the program you devise. The results may be tangible: Keep in mind that an estimated 60 percent of doctor visits are for stress-related complaints.

Other approaches beyond those cited can be invaluable, too. Some will come from friends, family, and your physician. In *Prescription II: Nurture Your*

Relationships, you were asked to examine your relationships with your closest friends and family; a sharing, caring relationship in itself can play a major role in managing stress. *Prescription V: Connect with Your Community* also relates, since the pursuit of meaning and purpose in life in a public way can enhance your sense of control and self-esteem.

No matter how much we wish to control our lives, life is change. To remain healthy, we need to change with it. Sometimes that means slowing our patterns to adjust to the aging process; sometimes it means adopting more aggressive exercise regimes to improve our cardiovascular health. But adaptability—let's call it flexibility—is also a personality trait that we all need to cultivate.

Be sensitive to what makes you feel like you are walking a tightrope. If it is multitasking, close your laptop while you are on the phone. If you feel like you need professional help, consult your physician and talk to a psychotherapist. Cognitive therapy is one way to identify behaviors and change them; talk therapy can also help you to change your patterns. Identify ways to ease your passage and do not hesitate to seek outside help.

Stress reduction should be restorative (and, according to several studies, it will help prevent colds, too). Understand that while no life can be all smooth sailing, neither is it necessary to feel forever at sea.

taking a deep breath

Every second or so, we inhale life-giving oxygen into our lungs; a moment later, we exhale unwanted carbon dioxide and other toxins. Respiration is involuntary and an essential, life-giving process. Just ask people with lung problems like emphysema, COPD, chronic bronchitis, or asthma. They will tell you that, whatever the cause, shortness of breath can produce fear, anxiety, tension, and any number of other symptoms.

Breathing is precious. The reverse of shortness of breath is deep breathing. Like clean water, the sunrise, and the affection of a friend, we should not take the simple joy of a chest-expanding breath for granted. A short session of deep breathing is a great way to reduce stress and anxiety, to shift your mood onto a new and relaxed plane. Deep breaths will bring more oxygen to your lungs and thus to your body, brain, and other organs.

The basics. Some call it an exercise; better to think of it as disciplined relaxation. There is no one right exercise for deep breathing, but here's one basic approach:

1. Find a quiet spot where you can sit or lie down comfortably. Rest one hand on your stomach, the other on your chest. Close your eyes.
2. Inhale slowly and deeply. Be sure that both chest and stomach rise as you fill your lungs with air.
3. Hold your breath briefly (try counting: *one thousand one, one thousand two* ...).
4. Exhale slowly.
5. Repeat the cycle. Breathe deliberately, perhaps five seconds per breath. If you do it a dozen times, the minute invested will leave you more relaxed and alert.

Some people find a longer session rewarding. Try setting aside ten or twenty minutes. Concentrate on breathing *slowly* and *deeply*. Try imagining yourself in a peaceful place: in a rose garden or lying on your back on a hilltop watching cottony clouds float slowly by. Other related relaxation techniques have proven valuable to many people, too, so seek out meditation or workshops in other modes of relaxation.

YOUR BEST STRATEGIES FOR STRESS REDUCTION

At the core of this chapter is a two-step prescription that requires that you employ your body and mind to ease the pressure.

Strategy Nine: Stress Reduction Through Exercise

Find an exercise regime that works for you and employ it regularly. See page 109.

Strategy Ten: Change Your Thinking

Have you identified strategies of rethinking your life in a way that enable you to take challenges in stride? For suggestions, see page 111.

Sometimes poems or prayers offer the advice we need; a moment of high stress may be just such a circumstance. The following lines from the Serenity Prayer, usually attributed to theologian Reinhold Niebuhr, can convey to the skeptic and person of faith alike how a certain critical distance in looking at our challenges can help us live a healthy life.

> Give us grace to accept with serenity
> the things that cannot be changed,
> Courage to change the things
> that should be changed,
> and the Wisdom to distinguish
> the one from the other.

PRESCRIPTION V

CONNECT WITH YOUR COMMUNITY

THIS CHAPTER SEEKS TO CONVEY ONE ESSENTIAL: CONNECTIVITY enhances health. Numerous studies have led to wide-ranging conclusions about the importance of social relationships to individual good health. I have seen it in my life and so have you.

On the darker side, the link between isolation and suicide was firmly established long ago, suggesting that, at the most elemental level, other people give us a reason to live. Each year new research appears, some from clinicians and epidemiologists, some from social scientists and psychologists. These researchers have identified ties between strong social networks and lowered risk of alcoholism, depression, and even arthritis. Postsurgical patients with caring people around them need less pain medication and recover more quickly.

It is a demographic fact that married people live longer. A study found that lonely older women have higher blood pressure than those who report they have people in whom they can confide their problems. Another found measurably lower levels of stress hormones in men who lived in supportive environments.

The message? Having caring people around you—or even just making meaningful contact with them by phone, via the Internet, or by other means—amounts to a special kind of health insurance.

※

As SHE APPROACHED her sixty-fifth birthday, Maggie had no particular desire to retire. "I had never given retirement much thought," she remembered later. "I felt energetic enough to go on for many years, and the idea of retiring struck me as ludicrous and depressing." She had hoped to continue working for the Presbyterian Church on a year-to-year basis, but on the day she turned sixty-five, she found herself retired, honored by her colleagues with a gift of a sewing machine.

I did not know her then—we met later—but I do know the sewing machine remained unused. Contrary to Dylan Thomas's advice, Margaret Kuhn chose not "to go gentle into that good night." After more than forty years of working to improve society from within such organizations as the YWCA and the national headquarters of the Presbyterian Church, she was determined to continue her work. A growing interest in issues concerning the elderly led her to found an organization called the Consultation of Older and Younger Adults for Social Change. Its original mission was to combat *ageism*, the segregation, stereotyping, and stigmatizing of people on the basis of age. The organization grew rapidly and soon adopted a new, more exciting name. She became an inspiration and a colleague to many of us concerned with aging.

Maggie Kuhn brought the Gray Panthers into being at a time when most people took it as gospel that the elderly should disengage from society as they approached the end of life. She countered that older people were a vital resource. She worked to ban mandatory retirement, and such restrictions have now been eliminated in most occupations. Her activist philosophy embraced elder rights and human rights, civil liberties, poverty, and pacifism. She became a lightning rod for criticism in some quarters, but she proved to have a great knack for getting media attention for her causes.

Maggie Kuhn ran her Gray Panthers for a quarter century before her death at age eighty-nine in 1995. In her typical style, just two weeks before her death, she joined a picket line with striking transit workers.

I would suggest to you that Maggie Kuhn is a model from whom many people, whether older or younger than sixty-five, can learn.

Engagement with Life

In *Prescription II: Nurture Your Relationships* (page 57), my subject was the closest of personal ties, namely those with your spouse, your children, siblings, dear friends, and others. In these pages, the topic is that larger sense of connectedness we get from relationships that are more distant—but that can be every bit as rewarding.

Even sociologists have trouble agreeing upon what "community" really means, but I will start with a faith-based community since it is almost self-defining. If you are a member of a religious congregation, you already have a grasp of its sense of common commitment, shared values and beliefs, and the desire for a shared identity, usually in a familiar setting (a church, temple, mosque, or other place of worship). That is one sort of community.

For people with or without religious faith, a sense of community can also be found in schools, neighborhood gathering places, clubs, historical societies, gyms, adult education classes, reading groups, bowling leagues, and yoga classes, and, when you think about it, just about anywhere three or more people gather for a purpose.

That purpose can be strictly social. That was John's story. He's a seventy-four-year-old retiree in California's San Joaquin Valley. He resides in the same small town where he's lived since he was a boy. The place has changed a great deal over the years, but he gets a reassuring sense of continuity on almost every weekday morning when he has a coffee at the same coffee shop. For ten years, he has shared a few minutes daily with one or more of the other regulars; the cast changes a bit, but there are perhaps ten core characters. Some he's known since childhood, others are relatively new arrivals. The conversation generally isn't especially profound, covering the weather, the fortunes of the baseball Giants, local politics, the day's headlines, and health issues. But this network of people, none of whom are best friends, provides these men and women with an everyday sense of contact with a world beyond the walls of their homes.

Service may be a component of community, too, a means of making the most of the thousands of extra days we've been given. Joan lives in a midsize city in central New Hampshire. She retired early (at fifty-seven) because she felt she had lost her edge as a teacher and, with thirty-five years in service, her pension would be adequate to support her. Even before her last day, she was looking for ways to stay involved with her community. A doctor friend told her the community hospital in town always needed volunteers. She started working at the information desk in the lobby but felt underutilized after the first week. A hospital administrator recognized Joan had something more to offer and, in a matter of months, Joan found herself in charge of scheduling the teams of other volunteers who manned it. Within a year, the hospital's head administrator asked her to help with another volunteer service, one that coordinates transportation for seniors for doctors' appointments. Joan likes what she does: She meets new people every day, and has helped hundreds and hundreds of people.

John and Joan each found a means of establishing a new engagement with life, despite changed work status. Such engagement begins with the individual; it requires self-awareness of skills and inclinations. A positive attitude about yourself and your life will foster healthy connections with others, both in intimate loving relationships and in day-to-day interactions with other members of society. Caring for others, whether it is offering emotional support or giving one's time and commitment, adds a dimension to life that can enhance longevity.

I have a few questions for you to consider:

Q: *When did you last do a good deed for a complete stranger?*

Q: *Do you engage with the world two or more times a week beyond your imme-diate home environment, not just grocery shopping, but talking, working, or oth-erwise making contact with people you don't know?*

Q: *Can you find the time to be of service two or more hours a week to people in your town or area who need help?*

Q: *How many of your daily interactions are with people who are more than twenty years younger or older than you?*

Connecting with others adds vitality; it can bring a new sense of purpose that enhances life and empowers you to seek personal growth, whatever your age.

Social Capital

An invaluable asset in the aging years can be what is called *social capital*, that is, the presence of community resources. These can be the friends, neighbors, coworkers, fellow worshipers, or almost anyone else who helps give us a sense of real purpose. We may meet them in the workplace, through our children, or simply within the fabric of our everyday lives. But some of the most important social capital is accumulated while we are making a contribution in other ways.

Social capital involves not wealth but self-worth. Volunteerism, part-time or temporary employment, second careers, and caregiving can be a means of adding vital links to other people. Perhaps it is a once-a-week stint at a soup kitchen. Maybe it is taking on the job of recording secretary at your club. It doesn't have to be through volunteerism; you don't have to take this broadening of your horizons so seriously that it feels like a full-time job.

Many people develop social capital simply through exposure to other people with whom they share something important.

In Okinawa, Japan, half a world away from the United States, there is a cluster of centenarians and even supercentenarians (people who've reached the ages of 100 and 110, respectively). These long-lived people, along with inhabitants of other notable locations with a high quotient of long-lived people, all share a key factor: a strong social network. Their lives are object lessons to us all.

Having a real purpose in life is in itself life-giving. The case of Kirk Douglas is informative (yes, *that* Kirk Douglas, the movie star). For fifty years he made movies. When a stroke at age seventy-nine left his speech impaired, he shifted his energies to community work.

He established the Kirk Douglas Theatre to encourage young actors. He and his wife, Anne, created the Anne Douglas Center for Homeless Women, a rehabilitation center for women with alcohol and drug addictions. He spearheaded a campaign to build playgrounds in Los Angeles to replace outdated and dangerous play equipment around the city. "We attended every inauguration—four hundred of them," he remembers. "It was gratifying to see the happy, smiling faces of our growing citizens."

That is the aging public man at work. The private Kirk Douglas has some wisdom to offer, too. "When I was younger," he says, "my sense of love was not very deep. I was too involved with my career." When, at almost ninety-two, he wrote of the people around him, he saw them differently than he had in earlier years. About his wife of more than fifty years, he remarked, "Growing older brought me closer to my wife. It was like looking at her for the first time."

His life has not been all accolades and affection. After his stroke, he passed through a period of depression. He realized that, for him, "Depression is caused by thinking too much about yourself. Try to think of others, try to help them. You will be amazed how that lessens your depressions. That satisfaction is priceless."

Such an attitude adjustment is not the answer to depression for everybody, but an engagement with family, friends, and community can be life-enhancing for the very old, the old, and those of us wondering at the impact of aging.

Borrowing from the life facts of Kirk Douglas's career, think of your life for a moment as a motion picture, a story with a beginning, a series of events and adventures, but an unknown end. If you were to make a trailer, what moments would you feature? What characters would appear?

Most important of all, how do you feel about the star, namely yourself? If you portray yourself in an honest light, do you like the protagonist? Has this character gained wisdom and admiration through the years? Has he or she contributed to the common good? Perhaps it is time.

Strategy Eleven: Invest in Social Capital

The goal is greater interactivity in a social sense. We humans are social creatures: interdependent, adaptable, and flexible. As a species, we have evolved in a world in which we must rely upon one another and, as individuals, the more we can contribute to bettering that world, the better it will be.

THE ASSIGNMENT. Two questions:

1. Have you made a difference in people's lives?
2. Can you think of a way of doing so?

SETTING PRIORITIES. If you are thinking about making a life change, here's some advice:

- *Find the time.* This is twofold: First, you must do the homework; second, you need to find the time in life to invest.
- *Make a list, then make the calls or send the e-mails.* Making contact is

essential: Talk to people, explain your interest, offer your services. Use any contacts you have—friends, family, coworkers—to gather intelligence.

- *Build your own—and your community's—social capital.* If your community isn't accessible, you can make it more so. Are there walking paths, gyms open to the public, bike paths, or mall-walking programs? If there are none, you can help initiate them along with your friends or the larger community. But, finally, the motivation has to start with you as an individual.

- *Believe in yourself.* Albert Bandura, a Stanford University psychologist, has described a behavioral phenomenon he calls *self-efficacy.* According to Bandura, the individual with a strong sense of efficacy will achieve a greater sense of well-being than the person resigned to failure. If you accept that something is beyond your control—say, "Oh, heavens, my memory is fading!"—then your fears may be realized, if only because you let it happen. A feeling of confidence, especially one reinforced by others around you, can deliver a sense of mastery throughout life. This power of self-efficacy has been studied by oncologists in cancer wards, in children, in the acquisition of computer skills by older people, and elsewhere. The message is consistent: In the face of challenges, a sense of self-efficacy makes accomplishments achievable and reduces the vulnerabilities to stress and depression.

- *Make a list.* Read the papers, talk to friends, listen to the radio for public service advertisements. Ask at local schools, hospitals, churches, charities, Meals On Wheels, and civic organizations. Almost certainly, they all have jobs that need doing.

- *Do it.* At some point you need to take the big step. Do not expect the appreciation to flood over you; you are doing this because it is worth doing, not for the thanks you get.

- *Give the gift you can give.* Your legacy is yours to shape, and now is the time to translate your desire to make a contribution into action. What do you have to give? Maybe it is time. Perhaps it's expertise: the retired (or retiring) accountant, marketing person, carpenter, and teacher are always in demand. Whatever gift you have to give, you will find that giving grows on you.

the society of cyberspace

Ask people under twenty-five about Facebook or MySpace; for their generation, such social networking websites are a given. They are the preferred means for talking to one's peers, even for those who attend the same school and live within a few streets of one another. And it isn't only the young who rely upon these sites. According to ratings published by the Nielsen Company, social networking now consumes more Internet time than e-mail.

All these sites are platforms; that's another way of saying they are meeting places. People come together in cyberspace, drawn by common interests or activities, classmates, business contacts, and friends of friends. These modes of electronic connection enable members to share job openings, news, ideas, business opportunities, gossip, and all sorts for information.

Once the province of the young, these online communities have evolved. At Facebook, which has more than 250 million members, the fastest-growing demographic segment is women over fifty-five. LinkedIn has an older membership profile, since its reason-to-be is to encourage registered users to create networks of people they know and trust in business. Gather.com has been described as an online space for the NPR crowd (a third of its membership is people in their fifties).

Choosing a network. You can use the world of social networking to enhance your connectedness. There's a large component of older people in the social networking crowd. Ask your friends where they gather in cyberspace and, chances are, they'll have a favorite place (keep in mind that people over fifty-five spend more time on their home computers than any other age group). Ask your family, too. And do your own searching, using your own tastes and inclinations. You'll find places to learn, chat, make new friends, renew old acquaintances, keep up with current ones, and talk about almost anything. These are forums for discussion, expression, and connecting. Politics, food, travel, pets, books, college allegiances, geographic origin, cars, games, art, theater, movies, or a passionate interest in almost anything can be the basis of a site—and a connection for you.

Many social networking sites are targeted specifically to people of a certain age. One of them, Eons (www.eons.com), offers games, humor, and groups devoted to the many special interests of baby boomers. Another, Senior City (www.seniorocity.com), is for people over forty only. Second Prime (www.secondprime.com) looks to provide advice on volunteerism, while Redwood Age (www.redwoodage.com) has an environmental bent, and Eldr (www.eldr.com) has lots of blogs.

Find one you like. Or more than one—nowhere is it written that you can't meet different people in different places, have different friends, and exercise different interests. The bottom line: Cyberspace is a place where nourishing contact can be made.

A New Stage of Life

Retirement is a word with many meanings. For some, it seems the end of the rainbow, the reward for a life's work, a doorway to ease and relaxation. Retirement offers the chance to explore hobbies and friendships, new and old, and to travel. It can be, in short, a liberation, a springboard to new experience.

For other people, it just feels like the end: the end of life as they've known it, of gainful employment, of a good income. For people forced into retirement by downsizing or illness, it may be an unwelcome surprise.

If you have the choice, think through the shape of your future before you leave the workplace you know. While retirement has long been seen as freedom from the obligations of work, in changing times lots of people see their post-career years as a time to take up other kinds of work they wish to do. The impetus can be yours: You can reorient the nature of your work. Perhaps your focus may be less upon achieving sales or other business goals. Instead, you may seek to have an impact on the life of your community or on individual lives. It is up to you what kind of retiree you will be.

Retirement has begun to evolve in American culture as our society seems to be birthing a new stage of life. The old hard line between work and retirement is softening. If society were like geology, you might say that the tectonic plates of middle age and old age have drifted apart, and a new social reality has risen in the emerging fissure. Call it proto-retirement or *ur*-retirement, if you wish; whatever the name, it represents a social sea change. Not that traditional retirement is not the right model for many people. For people who are able to do what they genuinely enjoy doing on their terms, retirement can make them happy and occupied. There is nothing politically incorrect about saying, "I'm retired and having a ball."

In truth, what is more important than what you do is whom you do it with—do you enjoy your cohorts?—and the satisfaction it gives you.

"the give-back revolution"

Many people are making career changes to foster a sense of personal and social renewal. One is Bill Gates, software genius, entrepreneur, and Mr. Microsoft, who in 2008 announced he was abandoning the pursuit of corporate profit for the philanthropic life. Today he administers the Bill and Melinda Gates Foundation, which underwrites initiatives in global health, agriculture, education, and poverty.

Gates is not alone. Many other members of his generation, some of whom sought to change the world in 1960s, are now looking for ways to improve it as they look to retirement. Writing of such humanitarian moves, *New York Times* columnist Nicholas Kristof called it "the give-back revolution." More than a few people are involved; it is a growing tide of baby boomers. A 2005 survey conducted by the MetLife Foundation in collaboration with Civic Ventures found that fully *half* of all Americans between fifty and seventy are interested in finding jobs that help improve the quality of life in their communities, most often in education and social services.

Even in the absence of Gates-size assets, you may be able to find ways to pitch in.

You can find ideas at organizations like these:

- *Experience Corps.* The stated mission of the Experience Corps is to "partner with schools and local community organizations to create meaningful opportunities for adults over fifty-five to meet society's greatest challenges." The brainchild of John Gardner, former secretary of Health Education and Welfare and founder of Common Cause, Experience Corps has programs in place in twenty cities across the nation. Check them out at www.experiencecorps.org.

- *ReServe Elder Service.* Established by two philanthropic-minded New Yorkers, ReServe seeks to connect experienced retired professionals with compensated service opportunities that challenge them to use their lifetime skills for the public good. Visit them at www.reserveinc.org.

- *Civic Ventures.* Founded in 1998 by writer and social entrepreneur Marc Freedman, Civic Ventures seeks to encourage experienced workers approaching retirement to redeploy their expertise to address serious social problems such the environment, education, health care, and homelessness. Consult www.civicventures.org and www.encore.org.

There is a growing literature, too, about making the most of career options at the traditional time of retirement. Such titles as *Don't Retire, Rewire!* by Jeri Sedlar and Rick Miners and *Retire Retirement: Career Strategies for the Boomer Generation* by Tamara Erickson offer strategies for thinking about putting personal passions to work, perhaps in alternative settings or on less demanding schedules. There is a new version of an old career classic, *What Color Is Your Parachute? for Retirement*, by Richard N. Bolles and John E. Nelson, which speaks to the pre-retiree, advising how to plan now for the retirement you want later.

What all this good thinking shares is a recognition that the conventional model of retirement at sixty-five is not what most people desire; rather, given some reorganization of priorities, proven skills can be adapted for meaningful pursuits.

The Second Career

Even if you are not ready to retire, you may be nurturing a desire to do something different, as were Mike and Michelle, husband and wife.

Both were thirty-two-year veterans at IBM when they got wind of a new program called Transition to Teaching. Recognizing the need for highly qualified high school teachers in math and science, Big Blue had created the program to enable veteran employees to pursue second careers in teaching. The corporate goal was to help meet the burgeoning demand for high-quality teachers (according to the U.S. Department of Labor, the nation needs roughly a quarter-million new high school math and science teachers every year).

For Michelle and Mike, the program offered a chance to remake their lives in a way that they could give something back to their community. Michelle had explored the option of teaching many years before, but this time her employer's willingness to underwrite tuition costs for retraining suddenly made it seem feasible. As residents of North Carolina, both were eligible for intensive teaching skills courses offered under the auspices of NC Teach, a program tailored to help a mix of people who had no prior education courses, including midcareer professionals, make the transition to teaching. A year of transition was required, including a three-month leave of absence, but both Mike and Michelle made the leap.

Coming from the workaday world of a large technology company, they have found they can help teach kids how interconnected the practical and the theoretical are. When students ask, *Where am I going to use this stuff?* they have real-world answers. The pay scale is less, but there are other compensations. As Mike says, "I remember the effect one of my high school teachers had on me: He opened doors I did not know existed. Physics came alive in his classroom. I'd like to have that impact on some of my students."

Strategy Twelve: Pursue a Second Career

If you are thinking about making a life change, there are many factors for you to consider.

THE ASSIGNMENT. As you look to engage your world in a new way, be sure that you:

1. Talk through your thinking with your spouse and other family members.
2. Make a plan that takes into consideration the short and long term (make the move because it suits you, not just for the sake of change).

OTHER STEPS TO TAKE.

- *Identify the work you wish to do.* At this stage of life, aim for something that will give you more than just a paycheck. The idea is to make a move that will give you a change—*and* a chance to help others change. Seek a job where you will use not only your skills but one that suits your personality and your interests.
- *Do the homework.* Your new career is probably more than a single phone call or e-mail away, so examine your skills honestly. If there are career assessments available, take them and think about the results. Look at the job market since, at any given moment, there are growth areas in the economy and segments that are contracting. Information technology, health care, marketing, education, and alternative energy are some current good choices. If you need to update your skills, get the training you need to be a better applicant. Take a course, sign up for workshops, or educate yourself.
- *Use the network.* Learn everything you can about the business in

which you wish to work. Identify good sources of information on the Internet, in trade magazines and papers, and other media. Develop a working knowledge of the business: Learn to talk the talk (every business has its jargon) and to identify the players (Which company is dominant? Who is the new kid on the block?). As you understand more, circle closer to your target. Talk to workers in the field that interests you. Get appointments with human resource officers and job placement counselors. Every conversation ideally should end with another lead to follow and a better understanding of the kind of job you seek.

- *Make a personal plan.* Calculate the financial ramifications of a career change. If you are leaving an assured salary for an uncertain income, make sure you have a strategy—say, a three- or five-year plan—for the future. You may be able to get education grants or scholarships; you may decide to use some money you had set aside for retirement; you may be able to claim tax breaks or credits for schooling or retraining. Put a sound strategy in place rather than taking a blind leap.

- *Sell yourself.* Do not hesitate to share your enthusiasm and energy as you pursue this new career. A future employer is being asked to make an investment in you. Your life experience, your skills, new and old, and your willingness to adapt and learn must persuade him or her that your passion far outweighs concerns about your age.

Ruminating on Retirement

Retirement can be a reward for a productive working life. For some people it is a long-awaited time of no alarm clocks, rest and recreation, a chance to be with friends and family, or to travel. Maybe you have looked forward to investing the practice time you know you need to shave a couple of strokes off your golf handicap, or to pursue that hobby for which you never have enough time.

For some people, however, retirement can feel like suspended animation. The symptoms can be unstructured time that seems to evaporate, a sense of idleness, boredom, even depression. This happens to all sorts of people, some of whom in their working lives were highly motivated and successful. As gifted a businessman and tactician as Lee Iacocca found that, after a few years away from the workplace, he felt as if he had "flunked retirement."

Of course retirement is not a pass-fail course, but there is good reason to educate yourself a little bit on the options and to try to suit your post-career life to your personality.

As our world has changed, the concept of retirement has evolved. When the Committee on Economic Security was tasked by FDR to devise a safety net to prevent poverty among "old people" who were "dependent" and "beyond the productive period," the average life expectancy was just sixty-one. Now the average American lives some seventeen years longer, and a number will enjoy that dividend of many more years beyond the old expectation. Today's retirement-age Americans expect to enjoy robust good health in the aging years, and they approach the transition not only healthier but wealthier and better educated than their parents and grandparents.

A benchmark survey conducted by AARP discovered something else that separates the generations: Fully 80 percent of baby boomers plan to work at least part-time during retirement. Part of this is a function of widespread concerns about financial security. The old joke about retirement accounts encapsulates the worry nicely. *How much money is enough to retire?* the jokester asks. The punch line: *No such thing.* That sense of economic concern grew by a magnitude with the financial uncertainties that arrived in the fall of 2008.

If the not-enough-money syndrome leads many people of retirement age to keep working in order to live comfortably, there is more to work than financial compensation. How about the Manhattan breast cancer surgeon who retired after more than twenty-five years in the OR but remained involved with patients, working in a clinic two days a week advising women at risk for breast and ovarian cancers? Or the teacher who, after thirty years in the classroom, mentors student teachers in her old school. One of the attractions of such jobs is the opportunity to stay involved with other people. Such work can offer a sense of purpose.

Some retirees make a point of avoiding the word *retirement*, afraid of its negative connotations. For them there is a stigma about leaving the workforce; when introduced to new people they're afraid "I'm retired" will be heard as "I'm old and not up to much." They do not want to be labeled with a stereotype.

Instead, they look to be consultants. Or to do volunteer work on a regular schedule. Coaching of all sorts, tutoring, mentoring, consulting, selling, making art, writing, and many, many other satisfying pursuits are out there. Again, don't be afraid of accumulating social capital.

rock of ages

The guitars and drums are loud, the rock-and-roll rhythm unmistakable. But the performers? Not a one of the eighteen-odd performers on the stage looks to be a day under seventy.

Sure enough, these men and women of a certain age are offering up concert renditions of tunes by the Rolling Stones, Sonic Youth, and the Talking Heads. The group—called the Young@Heart Chorus—first got together in 1982 in a housing project for the elderly in Northampton, Massachusetts. Since then Young@Heart has performed in Los Angeles, Canada, Australia, London, Rotterdam, and all over. In 2007 a documentary that records one season of rehearsals and performance went into theatrical release (it's called, aptly enough, *Young@Heart*).

As amusing as it is to see the gray and the gimpy taking on a tune by Radiohead, the genius of the organization is not entirely musical. And it certainly is not only about performance. The documentary reveals the camaraderie, the social support, and the challenges of rehearsals as these older people work to learn new tunes. As you watch them prepare for a concert tour, you see the individual strengths, the sense of community, and the sheer pleasure of singing. In a sense,

Father Time brings these oldsters together and, eventually, he takes them away (two members died during the making of the movie; none of the original members is still with Young@Heart). But the sheer joie de vivre, as well as the desire to push on and make more music, offers a bracing blend of humor, reality, and human sharing.

Not to mention the underlying message: As one undergraduate wrote after seeing Young@Heart perform at Dartmouth College, "It is possible to grow old without growing boring."

PRESCRIPTION V

TWO STRATEGIES FOR CONNECTING TO YOUR COMMUNITY

Strategy Eleven: Invest in Social Capital

Do something for yourself and your community. It will enable you to enhance your social connectivity.

Strategy Twelve: Pursue a Second Career

If the time has come to do something different in your work life, do the legwork and shape a new workaday life that gives back to society and offers you a chance for personal growth.

More interaction with your world can make your life more vital and satisfying *and* give you more reason to live a long and useful life.

PRESCRIPTION VI

LIVE THE
ACTIVE LIFE

THE HUMAN BODY IS CAPABLE OF REMARKABLE FEATS OF FLEXIBILITY, strength, and endurance. We can move with speed and grace, with stealth and agility. One of our great pleasures is sport in all its guises: throwing, catching, and hitting balls; swimming and walking; hiking, running, and climbing, in cold weather and warm, outdoors and in.

I find some people in midlife take the remarkable capacity of their bodies for granted. As we age, the fun we can have engaging in physical activity may diminish, yet that makes it all the more important that we recognize the essential role our physical condition plays in virtually every aspect of lives. Our ability to transport ourselves long and short distances, to prepare the food we eat, tend to our own personal needs, get the mail, take out the trash, make love, and almost everything else in life requires some level of physical function. Yet too many of us have settled into lives where we spend far more time sitting, watching, and driving than we do engaged in physical activities. Even when we are active, often we do the same things repeatedly, which is not always the best for our overall physical condition.

In the absence of regular physical activity, the human body rapidly loses mass as it ages. After age thirty, the bones begin to grow thinner, as the body uses the calcium and other minerals stored in the skeleton faster than they are deposited. This loss of bone density and strength is called *osteopenia*. In women after menopause, the process of bone loss accelerates. It may lead in women and older men to the severe demineralization of *osteoporosis* (see page 169).

Our muscles also diminish with age, losing not only strength but actually getting smaller, with the result that our ability to do physical work decreases. This process is called *sarcopenia*, and it is analogous to the bone loss of osteopenia.

I offer you a solution, one that can make a great difference in your odds of a healthy three-decade dividend: *It is a simple scientific fact that exercise can help maintain both bone and muscle mass.*

Your maximum heart rate also declines over time. During the aging years, that means the peak rate at which your heart can work decreases by perhaps seven or eight heart beats per minute in each passing decade. Lung capacity decreases with age, meaning less blood flow and oxygen delivery to the cells of the brain and other organs.

The preventative? *Both lung capacity and overall heart health are enhanced by regular exercise.*

As we age, our sense of balance becomes more precarious. The extra pounds that seemed like no particular burden in youth suddenly may make climbing a flight of stairs a demanding task. The risk of high blood sugar and type-2 diabetes increases over time. This is very far from a comprehensive list—*but these, and other changes that aging brings, can be counteracted, at least in part, by regular exercise.*

Lack of exercise plays a role in another risk factor in the young and old: overweight. The Centers for Disease Control estimates that more than 120 million Americans are overweight. As of 2007, only one state had an obesity rate of less than one in five; in the years since, the numbers have only grown worse. Across the population, roughly one in three American adults is obese, and it is no coincidence that exercise percentages closely track the numbers for overweight and obesity. An estimated 60 percent of Americans get too little exercise, almost 30 percent none at all. One does not have to be an epidemiologist to grasp the connections between such statistics. In an article I co-wrote for the *New England Journal of Medicine* in 2006, we rang a warning bell: Obesity is such a danger to the nation's health that the steady rise in life expectancy seen in the twentieth century appears to be slowing; statistical studies suggest that the youth of today may, on average, live less healthy and perhaps shorter lives than their parents.

In facing down the calendar, exercise can be an invaluable strategy not only in keeping you trim but also in reducing the potential impact of such risk factors as smoking and hypertension, too. The more frequently you find the time to get your body in motion, the greater the benefit.

The bottom line is even more dramatic: *New studies and old have consistently demonstrated that people who are active live longer than those who are sedentary.*

Strategy Thirteen: Determine Your Body Mass Index

The body mass index (BMI) is a means of measuring weight range. This basic assessment is an excellent place to start in evaluating your overall fitness. In average individuals, the body mass index is used to classify whether you are underweight, normal, or overweight.

MAKING THE CALCULATION. To perform the calculation, you need just two numbers, namely your height and weight. You can consult the National Heart Lung and Blood Institute website to do the calculation for you (see www.nhlbisupport.com/bmi), but you can do it yourself this way:

1. First, divide your weight in pounds by 2.2 (there are 2.2 pounds in a kilogram).
2. Divide your height in inches by 39.4 (the number of inches in a meter), then square your height in meters (multiplying it by itself).
3. Divide your weight in kilograms by the square of your height. For example, the calculation for a 180-pound person who stands six feet (72 inches) tall, the arithmetic runs as follows:

180 ÷ 2.2 = 82 kg
   [Your weight in pounds _____ ÷ 2.2 = _____]
72 ÷ 39.4 = 1.83 m
   [Your height in inches _____ ÷ 39.4 = _____]
1.83 x 1.83 = 3.35
   [Your height in meters, squared = _____]
82 ÷ 3.35 = 24.5 BMI
   [Your weight ÷ height squared = _____]

WHAT THE NUMBERS MEAN. Depending where on the scale your BMI falls, you may be classified as underweight, normal, overweight, or obese.

- *Underweight: A BMI less than or equal to 18.5.* If your number falls in the low range, that is not necessarily a good thing, and your health can be at risk. Low body mass can reduce your body's ability to fight infection and may lead to bone loss (osteoporosis) and decreased muscle strength and make it more difficult for the body to regulate your temperature. Talk to your physician to determine whether you should seek to gain weight.

- *Healthy weight: A BMI greater than 18.5 but less than 25.* People in this range are described as having ideal body weight. Statistically, they live longer with a reduced incidence of serious illnesses, and in most cultures are regarded as more physically attractive than those who are notably heavier or much slimmer.

- *Overweight: A BMI greater than 25 but less than 30.* Excess weight is associated with a variety of illnesses, including diabetes, cardiovascular disease, and hypertension. Weight reduction through diet and exercise is recommended.

- *Obese: A BMI greater than 30.* A person whose weight is 20 percent or more than his or her ideal body weight is classified as obese. If you fall into the obese range, you are at substantially increased risk for a variety of illnesses. The higher the BMI, the more urgent the need to adopt a weight-loss plan.

- *Morbidly obese: A BMI of 40 or more.* The morbidly obese person typically has a body weight of a hundred pounds or more over ideal body weight. Also called clinically severe obesity, morbid obesity is regarded as a serious chronic disease, with greatly increased risk of early death, heart disease, hypertension, arthritis, sleep problems, gastroesophageal reflux (heartburn), diabetes, and other disorders.

- *A word of warning.* Because this calculation is based solely on height and weight measurements, it does not directly measure body fat. Rather, the body mass index merely correlates with the amount of body fat in most people. As a result, the BMI may be misleading for certain people, such as athletes, whose BMI may classify them as overweight even if they do not have excess body fat (muscle tissue is more compact than fat cells, so dense musculature can skew the calculation). One easy way to be sure that the number you have calculated as your BMI is not misleading is to measure your waist circumference (see page 181).

fitness and fatness

Research has found that there is often an association between excess pounds and a greater risk of heart disease, diabetes, and other ailments; our society has found it convenient to accept that the inverse is also true, namely that slim people are healthier. The reality, researchers are finding, is more complicated.

In a study reported in 2008, the health of a nationally representative sample of more than five thousand patients was examined. Their blood pressure and levels of HDL cholesterol, triglycerides, and blood sugar were measured. Each participant was also classified as normal, overweight, or obese using the body mass index (see page 141).

The results were not as clear-cut as traditional wisdom might suggest. Roughly one in four of the individuals whose weight fell into the healthy range were found to have two or more risk factors for cardiovascular disease more usually associated with obesity. Conversely, roughly a third of the obese participants were found to be metabolically healthy.

Translation? Slim individuals are not immune to cardiovascular disease, and people who are overweight are not automatically at elevated risk. Body size is a useful but far from absolute indicator.

Getting a Workout

It is never too late: Exercise of the proper sort is good for you, whatever your age. If you have been active all your life, finding an age-appropriate means of remaining so is important, but even for people who have lived sedentary lives for many years, improving their physical conditioning can enhance their chances of longevity.

I especially like the story of the Wisconsin man who, at age sixty-two, was inspired by watching a marathon. He took up running, and, just a year later, ran in his first marathon, turning in the impressive time of three hours, twenty-five minutes (that means he ran twenty-six eight-minute miles in succession!).

The human body is remarkably adaptable, as one study of five thousand over-seventy adults found. All the participants already had some physical limitations, but those who got even minimal exercise (defined as the equivalent of walking a mile at least one day a week) were 55 *percent less likely* to develop more serious physical limitations (defined as severe joint pain or muscle weakness) that could compromise their independence.

Just as it is never too late, it is never too soon. The person who enters the aging years in good physical condition and who maintains a regular schedule of physical activity has a head start on longevity. If you have an exercise regimen, I recommend you stay with it. If you have drifted away for some reason, reestablish your ritual. If what you were doing no longer suits your health status, age, or inclination, there are plenty of other options out there; we will talk about some of them in the following pages.

We all benefit from healthy physical activity. Some people have a metabolism that seems to allow them to eat what they wish, exercise little, and maintain a healthy body weight. Often, however, that convenient illusion begins to fade during the aging years. The threshold at which physical decline begins is not reached all of a sudden; but in middle age and after, it is a fact of life. Being ready to push back is a good strategy.

A regular pattern of healthy physical activity will produce other dividends. Exercise plays a role in enabling our bodies to handle everyday stress. Exercise has been found to be as effective as selective serotonin receptor inhibitors (a class of prescription antidepressants) in treating depression. Exercise can lower cholesterol levels and, in some people, eliminate the need for cholesterol-lowering drugs. People who raise their heart rate and get the blood pumping vigorously through their bodies—and brains—have better cognitive function, too.

THE TRUE TALE OF TWO AGING TENNIS PLAYERS IS REVEALING. Trim, healthy, and competitive to the core, Brian and James are lifelong friends who have been passionate about the game since childhood. In their youth, they found tennis satisfied a basic need for competition. Each made his college team and, later, won his share of club and community tournaments. Tennis was a part of the fabric of their lives, and, through their forties and fifties, Brian and Jim played whenever they had the chance. Packing for business trips (Brian a salesman, Jim a corporate lawyer) meant tennis rackets as well as ties.

Good marriages produced children; the kids, boys and girls alike, were taught tennis. For each man, it had been a rite of passage when he lost to a son for the first time. Even now, more than twenty years later, Jim still shakes his head as if to clear the cobwebs when he thinks of the first time his daughter Sarah, then captain of her college team, sent him to the showers on the short end of the score.

More recently, a different sort of shock was administered not by a daughter but by Father Time. In Brian's case, it was recurrent knee problems that another arthroscopy could not fix; for Jim, there was searing shoulder pain that two surgeries hadn't cured. As another spring approached (along with the men's sixty-fifth birthdays), they found themselves pondering retirement from tennis. Age had been catching up, but could they, *should* they, retire their rackets? The two men reached different but considered answers and now, several years later, I think we can learn from their solutions.

Brian gave up singles. He found a tennis club where he could play on grass and clay; no more hard surfaces for him. He does not play as often and limits himself to three sets. He ices his knee immediately after playing, and takes off all days on which the joint feels wonky. He's taken up coaching a middle-school girls' team, which satisfies his urge for competition, and he cherishes the role the game has played and continues to play in his life.

Jim's doctor told him that he could continue to play but that he would have to learn to serve left-handed. He tried it a couple of times, but he hated feeling like a loser. Jim's not much for grays: It is black or white, play or not. So for him, retirement from the game was the only way. But he's moved on. He walks several miles a day and has found a friend to hike with once a week in the Vermont woods that he loves. It relaxes him, he finds, in a way that tennis once did. And his shoulder does not keep him awake at night anymore. Both men have made their peace with change and found different ways to satisfy their need to be active.

TYPES OF EXERCISE. Not all exercise is the same. Aerobic exercise seems to gather the most press coverage, but there are three other essential kinds of physical activities upon which good physical health in the aging years is built. Taking a vigorous thirty-minute walk at least three times a week is a safe and efficient means of getting the aerobic workouts you need, but for maximum health benefit, I recommend you consider not only your heart-and-lung conditioning but a broader exercise approach to enhance your balance, strength, and flexibility, too. Let me explain.

Aerobic Exercise. Running, swimming, and other sustained activities that raise your heart rate are termed *aerobic* (the term means, literally, "with oxygen," as this type of activity promotes the flow of oxygen to the cells). Not only does the heart muscle get a workout when doing endurance exercise, but aerobic exercise also helps keep the arteries elastic, promotes collateral circulation to the heart, and can help manage blood pressure. As usual, there are a range of corollary benefits, like burning excess calories and improved immune function. I find that regular aerobic exercise also elevates mood. (See *Strategy Fourteen: Select an Aerobic Exercise*, page 151.)

Balance Exercises. You cannot afford to take for granted your essential ability to maintain your physical equilibrium. The sense of balance begins to erode in the aging years; the result can be falls and fractures. But a few easy-to-do balance exercises are the single best preventative. Good balance also makes possible participation in sports, gives you better mobility, and builds confidence, so make sure you are working at maintaining your equilibrium. (See *Strategy Sixteen: Don't Take Your Balance for Granted*, page 160.)

Strength Training. To be sure you can still get out of your chair in the coming years—as many elderly people have found, it can become difficult—a few basic exercises can enhance the tone of your muscles. Strengthening exercises are important not only to build muscles but to prevent the wasting of muscle tissue. Muscles that are taken for granted cannot be counted on. (See *Strategy Fifteen: Strengthen Your Muscles*, page 156.)

FLEXIBILITY EXERCISES. Older people tend to experience more daily aches and pains. Aging muscles warm up more slowly; day-after stiffness in the joints seems more intense over the years. But the message your body is sending is most certainly *not* that you should avoid exercise. On the contrary, more of the right kinds of physical activity will lessen the discomforts and make you better able to remain fit and active. We tend to lose flexibility over time, too, the ability to bend and reach and turn and contort our musculoskeletal system to serve our needs and wants. Once again, simple strategies can be employed to keep us loose. (See *Strategy Seventeen: Keep Your Muscles Flexible*, page 164.)

OVERCOMING FEAR OF EXERCISE. I have conversations every day with people who have arthritis or obesity issues. In clinical settings, I see patients who are waiting for hip replacements. Whatever the particulars, these people share a common concern. They are asking themselves, *Might exercise do me more harm than good?*

True, a too-vigorous workout or an activity of the wrong kind can result in pain or injury (if you have chronic knee or back problems, for example, then a routine of daily jogging is probably ill-advised). That said, if you start slowly and sensibly, appropriate physical activity *can* produce health benefits.

If you have heart problems or other risk factors—you are over sixty-five, a smoker, perhaps, or you have diabetes, high blood pressure, a hernia, joint problems, or other nagging health problems—consult your physician before embarking on an exercise regime.

But try looking at it from the reverse angle, too: Inactivity is a proven recipe for a loss of strength, flexibility, balance, and aerobic health, which, over time, can lead to lost mobility and even the loss of independence.

A plan for health-enhancing physical activity can be tailored for virtually everyone. You may wish to consult a fitness professional who can plan a workout specifically for you. There are multiple choices out there. If your joints will not permit weight-bearing exercise, swimming or water aerobics may be the answer. If your stamina is limited, ten-minute workouts can still make a difference. Even if you have multiple health issues, the right regimen can actually help you feel better and may help you regain lost mobility due to disease, age, or inactivity. Exercise is also key to postsurgical rehabilitation and, in the same way, it can be central to helping you feel younger.

As clinical research has repeatedly demonstrated, exercise can contribute to your overall quality of life. In one study of some 350 men and women, aged sixty-five to ninety-five, over a six-year period, researchers found that the participants who walked regularly were *twice as likely* to age without developing physical limitations.

Significant benefit can be the result of modest regular exercise.

Aerobic Exercise

In the 1950s, David Smithson's neighbors recognized he was of the place—his family had resided in their rural Massachusetts town for generations—but they certainly did not understand his penchant for running. After all, despite being well into his forties, he was to be seen early in the morning (*even in the winter!*) running up South Street, across Carter Road, and, well, all around town. *Very strange*, people thought upon seeing him run by when they took out the garbage, loaded their kids onto the school bus, or just went about their daily business.

A quarter century later, David was still running when the rumor made the rounds that no marathoner had ever died of a heart attack. Even though the claim was soon revealed to be exaggerated, Smithson's neighbors began to understand that the promise of running was clear arteries, and *that* was appealing. No longer was David a lone eccentric, as the running mania of the time meant that a lot of other people began to be seen in shorts or sweatpants plodding around the town's streets and ball fields.

By the turn of the new millennium, jogging had become very much a part of the fabric of American life for people of all ages, and the message that regular aerobic exercise equaled cardiovascular health had become received wisdom. In the case of David's fellow townspeople, they had a proven paradigm who still paraded himself before them on a more or less daily basis. David did not run as fast or as far or as often as he once did, but he was still at it. He had outlived many who scoffed at him so many years before. Most people had long since ceased to shake their heads in confusion but now nodded in admiration when ninety-something David Smithson jogged past.

monitoring your heart rate

While almost any exercise is better than none, the best exercise involves elevating your heart rate. Your goal should be to get your heart pumping between 60 and 80 percent of your *maximum heart rate* (MHR). Your MHR depends upon your age.

For example, for a seventy-year-old, the arithmetic would go like this:

Step I:

220 − 70 = 150   150 *is your maximum heart rate*

Step II:

150 × .8 = 120
150 × .6 = 90   90 to 120 *is your target heart rate*

That suggests that during exercise, when you take your pulse the heart rate should be between 90 and 120 beats per minute. Do the math for your age.

During your aerobic workouts—three a week, say, at thirty minutes each—you should reach and maintain this optimum range.

Like other muscles, those of the heart grow stronger with exercise. Aerobic exercise is the best way to strengthen your heart, and the stronger it becomes, the higher your tolerance for stress and strain.

Getting aerobic exercise does not require that you buy a pair of running shoes and go jogging. In fact, it has become an accepted public health fact that intensive aerobic exercise is not for everybody—and it is not essential to hedge your bet on longevity. For a time, jogging seemed like the magic answer, but a growing consensus has emerged that, especially in the aging years, for many people the risks of jogging may outweigh the benefits. (The injury rate for walkers in their seventies is about one in twenty, while among the same age cohort, joggers' injury complaints, though many of them are minor, occur more than *ten times* as often.)

Do not misunderstand: If jogging gives you joy and your body does not complain, then I recommend you lace up your running shoes and go for a run. But for those not ready to run three miles, play three vigorous sets of singles, or play full-court basketball with President Obama, there are other approaches. The American Heart Association and the Centers for Disease Control offer common recommendations for a basic plan: You should exercise five times a week, perhaps walking briskly for thirty minutes a session (or substitute three twenty-minute workouts of more vigorous exercise per week). Those are the ideals. If you can fit them in, schedule two sessions a week of strengthening exercise, too, but we'll get to that soon enough.

Strategy Fourteen: Select an Aerobic Exercise

The first priority is to find something you enjoy. If disinterest or dislike accompanies your workout on day one, your resolution may fade quickly. Do not be afraid to try something new, but don't buy a three-month gym membership if you are unsure.

THE ASSIGNMENT. Ask yourself:

1. Do I want to be outdoors or in? In the great outdoors, walking, cycling, swimming, and jogging can be good choices. Indoors you could try out an exercise bike, treadmill, or step machine; all of these can get the heart pumping and work your lungs and blood vessels. Dancing and Rollerblading can be great fun, too.
2. How can I make the process as engaging as possible? Do not limit yourself to the sports we did in gym class all those years ago. How about tai chi or dancing? This is about activity, the more often and the more varied, the better.
3. Have I considered the potential for overtaxing my muscles and bones? When deciding upon a kind of exercise, consider the wear and tear your body has already sustained.

THE ACTIVITIES. The following are suggested activities, but by no means is this a comprehensive list.

- *Walking.* For many of us, a regimen of vigorous walking is a low-shock and highly practical form of exercise. The risk of injury is small, and, aside from comfortable shoes, no equipment is required.

Climbing stairs or hills will get your heart and lungs working harder. Walking can be companionable when done with family, friends, or fellow members of a walking club, but it also needs to be a little bit of work. How hard should it be? If you can converse with no difficulty at all, you are not working hard enough. On the other hand, if you are breathless and cannot talk at all, that is too hard.

- *Running.* Jogging has become widely popular for many good reasons: As vigorous exercise, it raises the heart rate into your target zone; it requires little equipment, not so much time, and delivers such pleasures as companionship, weight loss, and sleep enhancement. If jogging works for you, stay with it.

- *Swimming.* If less convenient than walking or running—not all of us live in clement climes or have easy access to swimmable waters—swimming is a nearly perfect form of exercise. It puts little stress on the joints, so many people with joint problems find swimming pain-free. (In comparison, a runner's body sustains countless shocks when his or her weight shifts to the lead foot; that stress, which can amount to thousands of pounds per square inch, can lead to back, leg, foot, and other problems.) When you swim, the buoyancy of the water absorbs your weight. You are working just as hard to make headway with your strokes, with none of the concussive impact of pounding the pavement.

- *Water Play.* If swimming is not your thing, how about water aerobics or even "water jogging" (think of it as power walking in water), both of which are low-stress ways of getting a workout for anyone, but especially for people with knee, hip, and back problems. The water serves to cushion the shock yet provides plenty of resistance for a good cardiovascular workout.

- *Low-impact Aerobics.* In a similar way, low-impact aerobics classes involve exercises that use large muscle groups in continuous rhythmic activity but limit the exercises to those in which at least one foot contacts the floor at all times.

- *Other opportunities.* Climb the stairs: The elevator takes you up, of course, but does not raise your heart rate. Doing errands? Park your car and walk between stops. Ride your bicycle to work and you will be doing yourself—and the environment—a favor. Remember that one of the most common observations among those who study populations of older people is that, on average, more active people live longer than those who tend to sedentary.

  * Going to visit a friend? Suggest that you socialize while you are walking. Avoid drive-through windows; get out of the car and walk on your own two feet. Buy a push mower for your lawn.
  * Go bowling, play golf, go rowing or canoeing, climb aboard an elliptical machine or exercise bike, work in your garden, or engage in other activities. Even moderate exercise has been found to have protective effects.

- *A word of warning.* If you are starting from scratch after being sedentary for a long time, begin slowly and work up, ten minutes the first day, then add a minute a day. Or maybe one week at ten minutes, the next at fifteen. Be sensitive to your comfort zone: It will grow over time, but if you feel dizzy or breathless or experience a sudden pain or sense of exhaustion, *stop!* Work up to a minimum of thirty minutes a day, or, better yet, forty-five to sixty minutes daily.

boomeritis

The demographic burst in births after World War II has long been known as the baby boom.

More recently, the term "boomeritis" has come into use among medical professionals to describe the epidemic of pains, aches, and injuries to the bones and joints suffered by the aging generation born in the years immediately after 1945.

The boomers heeded advice about the association between cardiovascular health and aerobic exercise—in the seventies, they started running with a vengeance, and many have remained active ever since. If better overall health has been one result, another has been the recent wave of mature or aging athletes arriving in doctors' offices with musculoskeletal complaints.

The boomers are not alone: Musculoskeletal injuries are now the number one reason for seeking medical care in the United States. Philadelphia orthopedic surgeon Nicholas A. DiNubile coined the term boomeritis to describe the miscellany of worn-out knees, aching backs, bursitis, tendonitis, stress fractures, strains and sprains, and other ailments that sports medicine specialists see every day.

Preventive Strategies. First comes the recognition that if exercise is good for us (and, yes, certainly it is), then there can also be too much a good thing. That's especially true when an exercise program focuses on just one sport. Consider *cross-training* (that just means variety). If you're a runner, try substituting a swimming workout once a week; if it's just tennis for you and you're finding that mighty serve is causing pain in your elbow, go for a run now and then instead of playing three sets. An aerobic workout complements a weight-bearing regime (and vice versa).

Overused muscles, bones, and joints sustain injury—and healthy boomers (as well as their parents and children) benefit from a thoughtful mix of activities in maintaining balance, strength, and flexibility.

the step counter

Walking is a normal part of life; even in our car culture, going most anywhere involves some walking.

And, of course, it is a great way of getting some of the exercise we need. Walking back and forth to the car probably is not enough, though. If walking is good, more walking is better.

Would wandering the halls of the mall be enough? Well, probably not, as studies have shown the average person takes about four thousand steps a day, and we recommend ten thousand per day (the equivalent of walking about five miles, depending on your stride) to maintain a healthy lifestyle.

How are you supposed to keep track of your walking? Taking the measure of how many steps you take is made easy with a step counter, also called a pedometer. You clip it to your belt (it is about the size of a beeper). Most models have digital readouts with easy-to-read screens. The device will work for jogging, too, if that's your exercise preference.

Your pedometer gives you immediate feedback, offering information on your activity level. It can also function as a reminder, a behavioral cue that may help motivate you to be active. The pedometer requires no calculation.

Pedometers typically cost between $15 and $30. Check out the International Longevity website (www.ilcusa.org/pages/get-involved/ilc-shop.php) to find a reliable model for sale at a discount.

Strength Training

The human musculoskeletal system makes us the upright creatures that we are. Our muscles and bones give us mobility, the ability to work, to feed ourselves, and to engage in physical activities. Our joints—effectively, they're cushioned hinges that connect the rigid network of bones—function because of paired muscles. Thus, your arm bends at the elbow with contraction of the *flexion* muscles, and the *extension* muscles straighten it.

Along with aerobic exercise, strength training is an essential component of any exercise program to keep the muscles at full function. It will help counteract the gradual loss of muscle mass and density called *sarcopenia* (literally, the term means *flesh loss*). The bone loss of osteoporosis (see page 169) has garnered more publicity, but sarcopenia poses similar risks for older persons. In older people, the loss of strength may manifest itself in difficulty rising from a chair due to a growing weakness in the muscles at the front of the thigh (quadriceps) and in the buttocks (gluteal muscles). Further diminution of muscle mass can mean the person is no longer able to rise from a bathtub or toilet. Dressing, bathing, and other daily activities can become more difficult. The early loss of bone mass, called osteopenia and, eventually, osteoporosis, means a loss of bone strength that can result in fractures. Two potential results of advancing sarcopenia and osteoporosis are disability and a loss of independence, which can also mean loneliness and isolation.

The inability to rise from a chair may seem unlikely, but it isn't a problem peculiar to the very old. An important New Mexico survey found that *half* of those over eighty reported such physical disabilities, but statistics also show significant loss of muscle mass in about one of eight men and one in twelve women under seventy.

Neither osteopenia nor sarcopenia is inevitable or irreversible. A substantial body of knowledge related to strength training in older adults demonstrates that real increases in strength can be achieved, even in very short-term exercise programs. The elderly can get better, and people entering the aging years can take preventative steps.

Strategy Fifteen: Strengthen Your Muscles

Strengthening exercises are a key to enhancing longevity. The potential gains of weight training are surprisingly immediate: Older people's muscles acquire not only strength but mass when even a modest regime of weight training is pursued. A regular regime of strengthening exercise can help you feel *and* look stronger.

THE ASSIGNMENT. There are many ways of working your muscles and bones. Try some of these, for example.

1. Check out the weight machines at a local gym, YMCA, or exercise center; or
2. Purchase a set of dumbbells or resistance bands (they're really just overgrown rubber bands) so you can work out at home; and
3. Devise a program following the guidelines below and try to work out three times a week on nonconsecutive days.

STRENGTH EXERCISE GUIDELINES. A good weight-resistance program will work different sets of your major muscles: the legs and hips, the shoulders and arms, the chest and back, and the abdomen. The goal is to develop the strength and size of skeletal muscles by a program that progressively overloads the musculoskeletal system. The best choice for you is one that is convenient and congenial to your lifestyle.

- *Plan your regimen.* A *set* is a number of *repetitions* of a lifting motion. Thus, two sets of 8 repetitions means lifting a weight 8 times, followed by a brief rest, then lifting it another 8 times. The load (weight) may be applied via strength machines at a fitness center, using handheld barbells, through elastic bands or tubes, or even using your body weight, such as by doing push-ups or pull-ups.
- *Be familiar with a typical strength program.* The American College of Sport Medicine recommends a minimum of one set of 8 to 12 repetitions. The task is to overload your muscles to the point of fatigue while retaining lifting form. That means you should reach the end of your ability to do another repetition well; it does not mean complete exhaustion, pain, or injury. If you complete your planned workout of, say, two sets and do not feel taxed, more weight is required. If you have to contort your body to complete the last repetitions, the load is too heavy.
- *Work out on nonconsecutive days.* Unlike cardiovascular activity, which can be performed every day, strength training should be performed two or three *nonconsecutive* days per week in order to allow your muscles to recover. Three times a week for strength training is enough.
- *Add sets as you gain strength.* Adding a second, third, or even a fourth set will result in additional strength gains; a fourth will produce maximal benefit. People in the aging years, especially people who are frail or over sixty, should start with lighter weights and perhaps a single set of 10 to 15 repetitions.

- *Mix it up.* Remember that the human body is designed with paired skeletal muscles. A balanced resistance-training program will put a load on your muscles coming and going by incorporating both flexion and extension exercises.
- *Consult an exercise professional.* If you wish, talk to a trainer to help you tailor the perfect workout. But keep in mind that strength training at an elementary level is neither difficult nor dangerous; it is, for all practical purposes, an efficient form of manual labor for which our bodies have evolved. Keep in mind that any activity that requires more strength than you use now will be of benefit to your health and reduce the likelihood and severity of both osteopenia and sarcopenia.

the key three

This basic program of three strengthening exercises challenges more than 80 percent of the body's muscle mass. It requires two handheld dumbbells, the weight of which should be determined by your capacity, which will be a factor of your strength and sizes.

Wall Squats. With a barbell in each hand, flatten your spine against a smooth wall. Your feet should be shoulder-width apart, the heels about 18 inches (a foot and a half) from the wall. Now, bend your knees slowly to allow you to slide down the wall until your thighs are almost but not quite parallel to the floor. Press upward to rise back up.

Chest Presses. Lie on your back on the floor with your knees bent and arms perpendicular to your body. With your elbows on the floor, point your forearms toward the ceiling with a dumbbell grasped in either hand. Now, slowly extend your arms, bringing the weights together directly over your chest until your arms reach full extension. Lower your arms slowly back to the starting position.

Single-Arm Row. Rest one hand and knee on a bench with the other foot on the floor. Your back should be bent so it is parallel to the floor. Allow the other arm to dangle, weight in hand, directly below the shoulder. Slowly raise the weight, keeping the elbow close to the body, then lower it, in a piston motion. After exercising one arm, switch positions and repeat with the other.

An ideal strengthening workout should consist of more than three exercises, in order that you use all the major muscles groups in the hips, legs, chest, back, arms, shoulders, and abdomen. You would do well to add others to the three described here, but these three are a good beginning. Start out with one set of 8 or more repetitions of each, but for maximum benefit you should work out to the point of fatigue. Over time, you can add second and third sets and perhaps additional weight. A full workout of these three exercises requires less than ten minutes and will help you build muscle mass and strength.

Keeping Your Balance

Frank was sixty-six and thought himself in fine fettle. His doctor told him after his annual checkup that his blood pressure was excellent for a man in his aging years; the blood work produced nothing of concern. His marriage, career, church, and volunteer work in his community made him feel useful and happy. As did his first grandchild, born the previous year.

He kept busy, often devoting the weekends to household chores. One Saturday that autumn he climbed onto a ladder to clean the gutters before winter, something he had done every year since they had bought the house more than twenty-five years earlier. Without warning—he just could not explain it afterward—Frank lost his balance. One moment he was on the ladder, reaching into a gutter; the next he was in free fall. Fortunately, he landed atop a dense evergreen hedge, which broke his fall and left him with only scratches and a sore shoulder.

An estimated one in three Americans age sixty-five and over sustain injuries in falls each year; like Frank, many of them do so for no apparent medical reason. Unlike Frank, some experience serious medical consequences, as falls are the leading cause of accidental death among the sixty-five-and-over set.

While medical conditions explain some falls—low blood pressure, vision problems, and vertigo that result from inner ear infections are common causes—the explanation among healthy people is often nothing more than a decline in the sense of balance.

We take our balance for granted, but standing, walking, running, and even sitting upright depend upon maintaining our balance. Our perception of depth and of spatial relationships is balance-related, too. Whether we are crossing the street or dancing the fox-trot, our sense of balance keeps us centered and upright.

Independent signals from our inner ear, eyes, and the musculature of the legs and back enable us to keep our balance. The central nervous system integrates this information. Ever notice how touching or holding something can improve your balance? The brain adds that data to the mix.

As we age, the rate at which the brain processes the signals slows; the coordinated response to visual, auditory, and other stimuli becomes less rapid, leading to a decline in both balance and agility (the ability to maintain balance when in motion). The process can be cyclical, too: A decrease in balance and agility leads to a loss of confidence, so we begin to avoid activities that require balance and agility, further eroding our abilities.

Strategy Sixteen:
Don't Take Your Balance for Granted

Aerobic and strengthening exercises will undoubtedly be of value in helping you maintain your balance and agility, too. However, improved balance can be enhanced by employing other specific, non-strenuous, and simple-to-do exercises. They do not take a lot of time, but the benefits can be important.

THE ASSIGNMENT. First we assess. The following is a variation on the Romberg Test, a standard assessment neurologists use to evaluate balance.

1. Stand erect, feet together, hands at your sides. (Do this next to a kitchen counter or a sturdy chair that you can use to anchor yourself if you start to sway.) Close your eyes.

2. What happened? The person with excellent balance remains upright and unwavering. The person whose balance is not quite so perfect may teeter a little but remains in place. The patient whose balance is seriously compromised will immediately begin to sway and, without the use of a steadying hand or other movement, might well topple over.

THE EXERCISE. To improve your balance, try these variations:

- *Stage* 1. Stand erect, feet together, with your arms crossed. Remain still with your eyes open. If, after thirty seconds, you are still in place and have not moved your feet or arms, move to Stage 2. If not, try again and repeat daily until you can consistently maintain a steady standing posture for thirty seconds.

- *Stage* 2. Repeat Stage 1 with your eyes closed. Again, complete thirty seconds at this level before proceeding to Stage 3.

- *Stage* 3. Position one foot directly in front of the other, with the heel touching the other toe. Cross your arms over your chest. Remain in the position, with your eyes open, for thirty seconds.

- *Stage* 4. Once you have mastered Stage 3, work on it with your eyes closed.

- *Stage* 5. Stand like a stork: With one foot on the floor, raise your opposite knee to hip level (meaning the thigh is parallel to the floor). Maintain the position for thirty seconds, without allowing the raised foot to touch the other leg or the knee to drop below hip level.

- *Stage* 6. Repeat the procedure outlined in Stage 5 with your eyes closed.

YOU GET THE IDEA. The goal is to improve your sense of balance by challenging it. There are lots of other ways of fitting balance exercise into your day.

- *One-Leg Stands.* At the bus stop, while you are waiting for someone, or when you have an idle minute: Stand with your legs shoulder-width apart. Extend your arms straight out in front of you, palms down. Now bend one leg at the knee so your toe points at the floor. Hold that position for five seconds (ten if you can). Repeat five times with each leg. Once you get good at the one-leg stand, close your eyes and master it that way, too.
- *The Bird Stand.* When brushing your teeth or hair, stand on one foot: It is an excellent way of doing double-duty. No time is wasted, and twice a day you get a balanced workout.
- *The Heel-Toe Walk.* It is a throwback to childhood: Remember placing one foot immediately in front of the other as if you were walking a tightrope? It is another good discipline. So is walking across a room on your toes, then on your heels. As your balance improves, try it backward.
- *Be Creative.* Do not limit yourself to these exercises. Invent others: Tie your shoelaces while standing. Try doing what the police ask drivers they suspect of consuming excessive alcohol: Walk a straight line. Find a vector to follow (tile, flooring, or other joint lines on your patio, along a hallway, at the mall, on a ball field that's not in use) and hew to it. It may take practice. If you get very good and have a safe place to try it, try doing it with your eyes closed or by walking the same line backward. Dancing of almost any sort is good. Tai chi, the gentle exercise practiced by millions in China and all over the world, is a graceful, dancelike discipline that has been found not only to enhance balance but also to slow the bone loss of osteoporosis, reduce

stress, enhance strength, and even lower blood pressure and cholesterol levels. How about washing dishes while you are standing on one
leg? All these activities will sharpen your sense of balance.

Staying Flexible

Harriet had back problems as a teenager. She was very tall for her generation (six-foot-one) and when, at age seventeen, she came in with back soreness in the middle of field hockey season, her pediatrician told her, "Tall
people have more backbone—and more back pain." But he also gave Harriet a simple regime of stretching exercises that she was to do before getting out of bed in the morning.

The doc suggested this: Three sets each of straight leg lifts (one at a time,
the foot barely lifted off the mattress); a second stretch in which Harriet
bought a knee to her chest and held it there (first she did one knee, next
the other, then both); and then pelvic tilts (with knees bent, she was to
lift her bottom off the mattress while pressing the small of her back downward). She held each of these positions for ten seconds each for 10 repetitions each. Sometimes she did one set, more when her back seemed a bit
sore, as in the last months of her two pregnancies. She always tried to finish with fifty sit-ups. Elapsed time? A bit more than five minutes. Then she
went about her day.

The little stretching regime proved to be lifelong advice. Forty years later,
Harriet remains active, and she still does her stretches every morning (on the
occasional day she does not, her back reminds her with a tightness
she rarely feels otherwise). Over the years she has had a few episodes of
back pain (carrying toddlers was tough), but none that required more than
a heating pad or over-the-counter analgesics (she swears by old-fashioned
aspirin).

When Harriet was in her thirties, another doctor told her that she should rethink the running regime she had recently begun. He told her, "Having had back pain, you know you are prone to back problems. The shock the back sustains with every stride is an unnecessary challenge." So now she hikes a little and keeps active in other ways. Her stomach muscles remain toned (those sit-ups help), which lessens the burdens of the back.

Harriet feels lucky, but she also recognizes the explanation: She's a pretty good listener, takes orders well, and understands that a little disciplined prevention has made a world of difference in keeping her flexible and pain free.

※

DO YOUR MUSCLES loosen up as quickly as they used to? Cold muscles tend to be less flexible and, as we age, easing that stiffness requires more time and attention. Our tendons, the cordlike tissues that link bones and muscles, become stiffer over the years and less able to tolerate stress; the ligaments, which connect the bones, lose elasticity. All of which explains why we feel stiffer. The gradual breakdown of the cartilage that cushions our joints does not help, as its deterioration makes us more prone to arthritis.

There is another factor that helps explain why many people complain of stiffness: It is not aging at all, but a lack of exercise. Many studies have shown that a sedentary lifestyle is the biggest single factor in lost flexibility.

Strategy Seventeen: Keep Your Muscles Flexible

As the cliché goes, if you don't use it, you lose it. On the other hand, a mix of aerobic, strengthening, balance, and stretching exercises can really help keep you flexible and feeling young. Stretching may be the easiest of these vital strategies to ignore, but a simple regime of stretching exercises may make you feel younger.

THE ASSIGNMENT. Try this:

1. Incorporate into your daily regimen a few minutes of stretches.
2. Every day focus your attention on your posture.

THE APPROACHES. The following are several lifestyle-friendly means of loosening up:

- *Start the day with a stretch.* Begin your day by waking up all your muscles. Before you rise from your bed, flex each muscle. Start at your toes and work upward. Tensing and moving those muscles gets the blood flowing.
- *Exercise your range of motion.* This is another way of saying flexibility: A full range of motion is full flexibility. As you go about putting your body into use each day, gently rotate your limbs and joints around their allotted orbits. Respect the restrictions your body imposes: Pain means *That's far enough!* Push the muscles until you feel them complain, but only a little.
- *Do some stretches.* Whether you are getting ready for the day or stretching out before a workout, ease into it. When you reach full extension in any stretch, hold it for ten or fifteen seconds. Then relax a moment before doing it again. Three repetitions generally are enough. When stretching your muscles, keep still with muscles and other tissues at full extension. Do not bounce, as bouncing adds unnecessary strain.
- *Practice often.* Do some stretching every day. You might also develop a routine in which you do a more elaborate series of stretches at least three times a week. Combine stretching with your aerobic or strengthening work—before *and* after. The cooldown is just as important as the warm-up.

- *Use heat.* There are lots of other ways to address tight muscles and joints, among them hot packs, hot showers and baths, and saunas.
- *Try yoga or Pilates.* A disciplined series of yoga or Pilates positions can be a great help; directly massaging muscles and joints can ease tightness, too.
- *Practice good posture.* Standing properly reduces stress on the back, hip, knee, and other joints; it also protects bones and can prevent injuries and even deformities. For the arthritis sufferer, the person with back pains, and any other aging person, it is healthy to stand straight, head erect, with your gaze directed at the horizon, not at the floor. Do not let your shoulders tilt forward in a slouch; keep them back and aligned. Tighten your abdominal muscles to pull in your tummy; tighten the muscles in your buttocks, too. This will flatten your stomach and help maintain the natural arch of your back. If your feet are splayed to the side, point them straight ahead. Your legs should align, with your knee the directly above your second toe; if your knee points in or out, practice keeping your hips, knees, and feet aligned. Maintain good posture when you walk. Practice in front of the mirror.

    If good posture feels uncomfortable at first, with practice it will begin to feel normal. It will help you distribute the weight of our body evenly, reducing stress on some joints, and help you keep your balance. It will also help you feel and look younger.

stretching out

Regular stretching will improve your range of motion and help keep your joints supple and flexible. It can help reduce the risk of injury, too.

In general, stretching is best done when your muscles are already warmed up. Try stretching after a warm bath or shower or after a little light exercise, like a walk or a short jog to get the heart pumping. Here are three easy-to-learn and easy-to-do stretches that you can do most anywhere.

Calves. Standing about a step away, place both hands on the wall. Bend your left knee while keeping the right leg straight. Lean into the wall, with your feet parallel, your right heel planted, and your legs and spine aligned. When you feel a stretching sensation in your calf, hold the position for ten to fifteen seconds. Return to an upright position, reverse leg positions, and repeat.

Hips. Sit upright on the floor. Bend both knees to bring the soles of your feet together. Place your hands on your ankles and gently pull your heels toward your groin. As you exhale, apply pressure with your elbows to the thighs, pushing them toward the floor.

Lower Back. Stand with your legs straight, the feet shoulder-width apart, your palms resting on your thighs. Bend both knees and lean forward. Curve your back to look down at your navel, tucking the tailbone under the pelvis. Return to a full standing position with your back straight.

After a few repetitions of these, your muscles should feel warm and loose.

Going the Distance

Little more than a generation ago, the marathon was regarded as the ultimate athletic challenge and the province of the few. Those who ran it were young, regarded by many as slightly crazy, and entirely male (women were forbidden; women were then thought too fragile for the marathon or, for that matter, any race over two hundred meters).

Today, the competitors in a marathon consist of more than an elite group of athletic supermen. More women than men finish marathons in America; amazingly, people in their nineties complete the 26 miles and 285 yards. On average, today's marathoner is older and a bit slower than in the past, but the population of runners has exploded (during the late seventies running boom, some 25,000 Americans annually completed a marathon; today more than twenty times as many finish each year).

The marathon has become more than a race. The very idea of a marathon has become a metaphor for setting a goal and achieving it. To some, it is about success. For others, it is survival: Among cancer patients and docs, the marathon metaphor stands for life itself. You rise to challenges, you race, you survive. Life is not easy; rarely do the good things come easily. Toughness, planning, desire, discipline, and the exercise of sheer will are required.

Now, do not misunderstand: I am not recommending that everyone in the aging years take up distance running. But use the metaphor: Sometimes it is healthy indeed to aim at a goal, even a forbidden one, and achieve it.

For the marathoner and the novice walker alike, the first assumption is the same. You need to find the time and the initiative to get regular workouts. Inertia and life's obligations may make it seem impossible. In going about your life, you may already feel like the overworked student with no free periods, as work, family, community, and other commitments consume your day. Somehow, though, you need to push the distractions aside. Think of it as opening the curtains on a sunny day. There is benefit for mind, body, and spirit. You do not have to embark upon the perfect, multiphase exercise program involving a carefully calibrated mix of aerobic, strengthening, balance, and flexibility exercises. But it is in your interests to find the time to pursue at least some physical activity.

Look for exercise opportunities. Remember, you do not have to work out every day; a healthy minimum is a thirty-minute workout, three times a week. How about ten-minute vigorous walks, times three, on each of three days per week? Taking smaller bites of the apple may be a good way to make a little progress, feel a little lift, and to gain the sense that you *can*, that you *must*, that you *want* to do more.

At the very least, take advantage of the everyday opportunities you encounter. Opt for climbing the stairs instead of taking the elevator or escalator. Park at the far end of the parking lot. Do balancing exercises when standing in line at the airport. Use the carry basket instead of the cart if you are buying a manageable number of items at the grocery store. Do some housecleaning, rake leaves, work in the garden, wash the storm windows.

Physical activity is central to the goal of longevity. Give it a chance.

Osteoporosis

A loss of bone strength is a normal part of aging (the human metabolism begins to shed more bone than it builds starting as early as your thirties). When bone loss becomes excessive, it is termed *osteoporosis* (literally, porous bones), a medical condition in which the risk of bone fracture is increased.

Osteoporosis is more likely to occur in women after menopause. Thin people with delicate bone structure, low overall body weight, and those with a family history of osteoporosis are also at greater risk of bone loss, as are Caucasian, Asian, and Latino peoples. Patients subject to long periods of bed rest lose bone density, too, as do those who use certain medications such as the anticonvulsant phenytoin (Dilantin), corticosteroids, the blood thinner heparin, and the anticancer drug methotrexate. Women are about twice as likely as men to sustain an osteoporotic fracture in the later years, though after age seventy-five, the risk for men increases substantially.

UNDERSTANDING BONE DENSITY. The space program taught us something important about how our bodies use bone minerals. Space researchers observed that at zero gravity astronauts' bones began to "unload." The number of bone cells decreased, and the bones lost some of the minerals calcium and phosphorous deposited there. The skeleton thus weakened, the potential increased for now brittle bones to fracture. Doctors also observed that astronauts' bodies upon returning to earth began to regain lost minerals in their bones as soon as weight-bearing exercise was resumed; simply being subject to earth's gravitational pull initiated the restoration of calcium.

Osteoporotic bone is less dense. While the normal body both builds and destroys bone by depositing or removing calcium salts, withdrawals exceed deposits in the osteoporosis sufferer. With less calcium, the bones are weaker;

in severe cases, a slight blow, a fall, or simply lifting an object are acts that can result in breakage.

Of the 206 bones in the human skeleton, some are more prone to osteoporosis than others. The vertebral bones of the spinal column, the ends of the thigh bone (at the knee and, in particular, the hip), and the arm bones at the wrist are especially susceptible to bone loss. Minor vertebral factures can occur unnoticed, though sometimes a dull, nagging pain accompanies what are called compression fractures. Multiple compression fractures over a period of years are responsible for the loss of body height and the bent-over postures sometimes called dowager's hump.

Hip fractures are common among the elderly (some 350,000 older people annually) and are a major cause of disability and even death. Often hip fractures are the result of falls, although in people with advanced osteoporosis, less violent events can result in a break. Surgical repairs of hip fractures are now commonplace, and the procedure usually restores mobility and near normal function. However, surgical complications, the stress of the surgery, and the event itself can result in premature death (according to one recent study, almost 30 percent of older people who suffer hip fractures die within a year).

The least serious of the common fractures among those with osteoporosis is breakage of the larger of the lower arm bone, the radius. Such wrist breaks, called Colles' fractures, often occur as the result of falls. Typically the prognosis for regaining full function is good. The occurrence of a Colles' fracture is often the first warning sign of osteoporosis.

consume with care

Caffeine, alcohol, sugar, and salt have been called the "bone thieves." While there is disagreement among researchers as to a direct cause-and-effect relationship, it is likely that excess consumption of these food substances will result in reduced calcium absorption by your body.

Soft drinks, with their high phosphorus content, are also believed to rob the bones of calcium.

Wheat bran blocks absorption of calcium, so avoid eating it within two hours of consuming your calcium supplement.

Excess consumption of alcohol reduces bone formation and interferes with the body's ability to absorb calcium. Limit your alcohol consumption: for women, that's a maximum of one drink per day, for men two or fewer.

Prevention and Treatment. Today doctors do more screening, recognize warning signs earlier, and women and men in their aging years can employ preventative strategies sooner. Better treatments are being marketed, too. There is increasing hope that bone loss can be reversed, strengthening bones and restoring function.

The single best preventative is strong bones, which are best established before age thirty by consuming a diet rich in calcium and vitamin D, getting regular weight-bearing exercise, and avoiding tobacco and excess alcohol consumption. Not surprisingly, perhaps, the same strategies, as well as a number of others, are helpful in later life, too, as the risk of osteoporosis increases. I would advise that you take the following precautions:

Eat a healthy diet. A balanced diet is step one, since a mix of nutrients, among them vitamins K, B_6, B_{12}, and magnesium are important to healthy bones. In particular, emphasize good sources of calcium (especially milk, leafy green vegetables, legumes, green beans, lettuce, and calcium-fortified orange juice, especially for those who are lactose intolerant). Get plenty of vitamin D, too, by eating fortified dairy products, eggs, liver, and saltwater fish.

Live an active life. Exercise is essential, especially weight-bearing exercise (sedentary people, or those confined to bed for long periods, experience bone loss). Good weight-bearing exercise includes walking, jogging, dancing, and other activities in which your muscles work against gravity, as the pull of muscles helps build bone.

Use supplements sensibly. Food sources are best for both calcium and vitamin D, but in the aging years, in order to make sure you have a sufficient supply of both nutrients, you may wish to also take supplements by mouth. A daily multivitamin may provide what you need. A daily dose of 700

IU of vitamin D3 is recommended, along with two doses (600 mg each) of calcium taken at morning and night.

Quit smoking. As always, tobacco poses a health risk: Female smokers tend to reach menopause earlier, and tobacco may also have an effect on the body's ability to use vitamin D to absorb calcium.

Get screened. Your physician may recommend a screening test after age sixty-five or if he or she suspects osteoporosis. A bone mineral density test is the best means of determining the health of your bones. Today, the most widely recognized test is the DEXA (dual-energy X-ray absorptiometry). You will experience no discomfort as the X-ray is directed at the hip or spinal area.

Prevent falls. It is a given that falls pose a major risk factor for osteoporotic fractures. Recent clinical studies have found that conditioning, balance-enhancing, and muscle-building exercises reduce the risk of falls by approximately 25 percent.

Get some sun exposure. Since sunlight enables your body to make its own vitamin D, exposure to the sun is important, too. Ten to fifteen minutes three times a week is sufficient.

Look into medications. Osteoporosis is difficult to reverse, but your physician may prescribe hormone replacement therapy, a hormonelike drug called Evista, or one of the osteoporosis medications that inhibit the cells that break down bone and slow bone loss (Actonel, Boniva, and Fosamax are three brand-name drugs). A hormone called calcitonin is also prescribed to inhibit bone loss, and a number of new drugs are being tested and marketed, including a synthetic form of parathyroid hormone called Fortéo, which may increase bone mineral density. Each of these medications has potential side effects, so discuss the balance of benefits and risks of any drug regimen with your physician.

What Is Arthritis?

Arthritis is actually not one but many ailments—there are more than 150 kinds of arthritis—but each involves aching joints (the word "arthritis" comes from the Greek *arthron*, for joint, and *itis*, meaning inflammation). The most familiar varieties are osteoarthritis, rheumatoid arthritis, and gout (aka gouty arthritis), but other all-too-common types include ankylosing spondylitis, systemic lupus erythematosus, polyarteritis, and progressive systemic sclerosis. Each can interfere with your ability to live an active life.

In order to understand joint problems, I suggest you think of your joints as junctions where two bones (or more) are connected in a way that permits each to move in relation to the other. Fitted to the end of each bone is a cap of smooth white *cartilage*, a very tough tissue that acts like a sponge, preventing bone-to-bone rubbing and consequent wear when the joint is in use. A liquid called *synovial fluid* both lubricates and provides nutrients to the cartilage. It is sealed in the joint by the *synovial membrane*, which in turn is protected by a fibrous layer called the *capsule.*

When each of the body's sixty-eight joints is working correctly, we barely know they are there; on the other hand, each variety of arthritis reduces the normal function of the involved joint or joints. In the case of *osteoarthritis*, the cartilage becomes worn or cracked to the degree that it fails to cushion movement of the joint. In *rheumatoid arthritis*, the synovium periodically becomes inflamed. In the case of *gouty arthritis*, crystals formed from excess uric acid in the body accumulate in the synovial fluid; when the body, sensing something is amiss, attempts to rid itself of the crystals, pain and inflammation results.

The mechanisms for each type of arthritis differ, as do the treatments. Some require significant medical interventions—surgeries, daily medications, joint protection (walkers, canes, or splints), and adaptations to life patterns (changes in exercise, weight loss, physical therapy). Your family physician or, if appropriate, a medical specialist called a rheumatologist will guide your treatment. For most people with osteoarthritis, lifestyle adjustments rather than more radical interventions will enable you to remain active and engaged.

OSTEOARTHRITIS. By far the most common type of arthritis, osteoarthritis is among the most frequent disorders affecting the human race. It has been around since prehistory, as signs of the ailment have been observed in the mummified skeletons of the Egyptian pharaohs.

About fifty million Americans have been told by their doctors they have some form of osteoarthritis. (In comparison, RA affects about one in a hundred persons.) Countless others may well have joint deterioration of which they are blissfully unaware, since many patients with osteoarthritis first hear about it when their doctors tell them. It is commonplace for doctors to observe signs of arthritis when examining X-rays or scans ordered for some other diagnostic purpose. Osteoarthritis is also referred to as *degenerative joint disease* or *wear-and-tear arthritis*.

The pain of osteoarthritis begins at one location, most likely in the knees, neck, hips, lower back, or fingers. As the cartilage in a joint deteriorates over time, it loses elasticity or becomes frayed, cracked, or pitted, or even disappears altogether. With the breakdown of cartilage, the joint is more likely to be bone-on-bone, causing bone tissue to grate and gradually wear away. Bone spurs tend to develop at the edges of the joints, one of the signs that your doctor will look for in images taken of your joints.

There are three common categories of osteoarthritis. The first (and least serious) involves only the fingers. The joints become knobby, typically with bone spurs between the last two bones in the fingers, which usually develop over a period of years. Called Heberden's nodes (after the English doctor who first commented upon them), these lumps are usually painful at first, but the pain tends to disappear over a period of months. Women are much more likely than men to develop Heberden's nodes, which often recur from one generation to the next.

Osteoarthritis in the back and neck occurs when bone spurs develop on the vertebral bodies located on either side of a degenerated or collapsed disc. Sometimes impact injuries have preceded the appearance of the arthritis. Characteristic symptoms are pain and stiffness.

The third kind of osteoarthritis occurs in the weight-bearing joints, particularly the hip and knee. Osteoarthritis of the hip can be disabling, producing pain in the groin, bottom, the side of the hip, and the thigh, sometimes reaching downward to the back of the knee. A progressive loss in range of motion may also result. If not universal, such osteoarthritis is widespread: One recent study found that almost half of all Americans will develop painful knee arthritis in their lifetimes; among the obese, the rate will be closer to two out of every three.

Prevention and treatment. Arthritis is less likely to occur in people who maintain a normal weight, eat a healthy and well-balanced diet, and exercise sensibly to preserve good muscle tone and bone density. Joint overuse is a risk factor for arthritis (thus the retired ballerina with arthritic ankles and the former baseball pitcher with the sore shoulder), as is traumatic joint injury (the football player with the reconstructed knee is a likely candidate for osteoarthritis later in life).

Once arthritis sets in, however, there are many strategies for managing the pain and maintaining joint movement and health.

Medications. The shelf at the pharmacy that holds the arthritis remedies is a long one, with choices that range from household aspirin to narcotic pain relievers, from corticosteroids to chemotherapies also used in treating cancers. Some medicines are topical (applied directly to the skin), some are taken by mouth, others injected.

Your physician is your best guide to this pharmacopeia, but the most basic of arthritis pain relievers are the NSAIDs (nonsteroidal anti-inflammatory drugs), which can ease both the pain and inflammation due to arthritis. These include over-the-counter generics like aspirin, ibuprofen, and naproxen, as well as many prescription and brand-name drugs. If you feel you need more than occasional relief, talk to your doctor, since there are a number of side effects common to long-term use, in particular stomach problems, even with the over-the-counter medications.

Supplements. Pharmacies, health food stores, and supermarkets have a vast array of medicaments made from roots, leaves, stems, animal tissues, and synthesized in laboratories. These supplements—vitamins and herbs, pills, powders, or liquids—often come with bold claims of their efficacy. For the most part, supplements remain in the realm of the untested, but some do show promise. An early test on a pineapple derivative called bromelain found it reduced the discomfort of osteoarthritis in a way comparable to the NSAIDs.

Chondroitin sulfate, derived from animal tissues, has been found in studies to reduce inflammation and pain in the joints, as has devil's claw, a traditional herbal plant long used in Africa, and glucosamine, a component of cartilage derived the shells of lobster, crab, and shrimp. Fish oil has some effectiveness in rheumatoid arthritis patients. SAMe (S-adenosylmethionine) is sold as a drug in Europe (it's a chemical that occurs naturally in the body) and has been found in studies to enhance joint health. In general, however, be wary of any claim that seems too good to be true. Advise your doctor if you are considering the use of such supplements.

Exercise. Follow your doctor's advice, but recent research has shown that moderate physical activity three or more days a week helps relieve arthritis pain and stiffness. (Too little exercise can result in stiffer joints, a loss of muscle strength, and even disability as movement becomes more difficult.) Maintaining muscle strength with appropriate exercise is important, and regular physical activity will also make you feel more energetic and even lift your mood.

Moderate physical activity is recommended (activity that produces a slight increase in heart rate and breathing), and low-impact activities work best for people with arthritis (such as walking, swimming, riding a bicycle, and dancing). If you have a form of arthritis that is characterized by flare-ups, it is important to recognize when the pain and inflammation are most active and, during those times, to restrict your activity to simple range-of-motion exercises, carefully moving the joint as far as it can go.

A prescribed program of physical therapy may be appropriate, too. The goal is simple: Flexibility and strength are to be maintained or restored, but with careful regard for the weakened joints in order to protect them from further damage. A mix of flexibility and strengthening exercises should become a part of your daily routine.

Weight control. Carrying excess weight around puts additional pressure on joints and bones (that spare tire is really hard on the back), so aim to reach your ideal weight if you are overweight (see *Strategy Thirteen: Determine Your Body Mass Index*, page 141). The effects of weight control have been demonstrated by investigators: One study showed that women who lost as few as eleven pounds cut their risk of developing knee osteoarthritis and its accompanying joint pain in *half.*

Joint protection. People who experience sports injuries or have jobs with repetitive motions like repeated knee bending are more likely to have osteoarthritis; once the arthritis strikes, steps can be taken to avoid exacerbating joint injury or soreness.

For many people with sore joints, a few basic commonsense rules may help, too. For example, use large joints where possible to perform a task (open a door with your arm instead of just your hand). Distribute the weight over several joints when lifting something; use two hands rather than one in moving even small objects. Move your joints naturally, avoiding awkward, overreaching, or uncomfortable movements. And most of all, listen to your body: Do not make your joints do things your body is warning you that you should not ask of them. In some cases, walkers, canes, or splints may be appropriate.

Surgery. One of modern medicine's great strengths is in correcting mechanical problems, and joints are as mechanical as the human body can get. Joint replacements, called *arthroplasties*, are now everyday procedures, used to replace all or portions of knee, hip, shoulder, finger, and other joints. In general, however, surgery is appropriate for more serious cases, and less radical treatments such as exercise, pain control, stress management, and perhaps weight loss are preferred. If, however, your hip, knee, or another joint is causing constant pain; if it is limiting your ability to get into a car or climb stairs; and/or it is awakening you at night, substantial improvement in your condition may be gained by replacement of the damaged joint.

YOUR FIVE STRATEGIES TO BETTER PHYSICAL CONDITION

As you plan for longevity, you need to integrate aerobic, strengthening, balance, and flexibility exercises into your life.

Strategy Thirteen: Determine Your Body Mass Index

This will give you a framework for thinking about an exercise program (see page 141).

Strategy Fourteen: Select an Aerobic Exercise

Find an exercise routine that you can follow three or more days a week, twenty to thirty minutes per day (such as walking, running, or swimming; see page 151). If that's too difficult for you, try two or three ten-minute sessions per workout day.

Strategy Fifteen: Strengthen Your Muscles

At least two times a week perform some type of strength training, whether you use a weight machine, a free-weight program under the guidance of a professional trainer, or the Key Three for a compact and sensible workout (see pages 156 and 158).

Strategy Sixteen: Don't Take Your Balance for Granted

Employ the Romberg variations at least three times a week to tune up your sense of balance (see page 160).

Strategy Seventeen: Keep Your Muscles Flexible

Find a few minutes every day to stretch taut muscles and joints—in the morning, at bedtime, or before and after workouts. Or use the trio of stretches described in *Stretching Out* (see pages 164 and 166).

Incorporating regular physical exercise into your life can be invaluable in controlling weight and maintaining flexibility, mobility, and even maximum cognitive function.

PRESCRIPTION VII

EAT YOUR WAY
TO HEALTH

❖

EATING IS ONE OF LIFE'S INDISPUTABLE JOYS. NOT ONLY DOES food sustain us by providing the fuel we need to function, it enables us to be social beings, to break bread with friends and family in common repast. Certain meals come complete with important ritual and religious significance. The foods we share with others can convey our status; the foods we consume on our own may offer us comfort or solace. Most of all, the taste, texture, and aromas of our favorite foods please our palates as they fill our stomachs.

I don't think for a moment that life is supposed to be about deprivation, and certainly this book is not. Our pleasures help make life worth living, and I am not about to tell you that you should go about starving yourself as you make the most of your dividend years. On the other hand, a long life depends in part on good decisions about how we live our lives, and nowhere is that more true than when it comes to our dining pleasures.

Eating the wrong foods—or even eating too much of the right ones—can play a role in heart disease, the leading cause of death in the United States. The foods we eat may dispose us to stroke, diabetes, high blood pressure, certain cancers, osteoporosis, and other ailments. In contrast, some foods enhance digestion, buttress the immune system, and can help us maintain a healthy weight.

Nutrition's role as a major determinant of the life course is suggested by the story of a pair of twins. Scientists delight in circumstances like theirs, which offer insight into the ongoing nature-versus-nurture debate. Separated as children, the two boys went in different directions at age nine when their parents died in an automobile accident. Joshua went to live with his grandparents in the newly founded nation of Israel. He subsequently served in the Israeli army, married, and as a young man went to live on a kibbutz, where he raised a family. His relationship with the land is reflected in his diet: ample fresh fruits and vegetables at every meal, local yogurt, and whole-grain breads made in the community bakery of wheat grown in nearby fields. He eats more fowl than red meat (in fact, Josh operates an ostrich farm). Today he is sixty-eight, weighs roughly what he did at age twenty-one, and remains in excellent health.

His brother, Jonas, lived a different life. He remained in America with an uncle, attended American colleges, and became a successful businessman. He lived in suburban New York, married, had children, and by most standards lived a happy and reasonably healthy life. He ate the standard fare for upper-middle-class Americans in his time, which amounted to lots of meat and potatoes. His job was stressful, his commute into New York City was time-consuming, and he was taking a daily pill for high blood pressure by the time he was forty-five. When he died of cardiac arrest at age sixty-one, he was about forty pounds overweight.

Diet and disease, cause and effect? Science rarely sees things in such stark black-and-white terms. But the lifestyle differences are revealing and provide food for thought. The story also illustrates once again that genetics are far from the sole determinant of longevity.

Keep in mind that for many people, moderate dietary adaptations can reduce insulin levels, blood pressure, blood cholesterol, and triglycerides, as well as overweight, all of which are significant factors in the aging process. *That means you can eat your way into feeling and looking younger.*

waist circumference

Like the body mass index (see page 141), the waist circumference is a useful health indicator. Many ailments are associated with obesity and, since we tend to carry fat around our waists, this simple measurement can be very telling.

To determine your waist circumference, position a measuring tape around your middle at the upper hip bones; make sure the tape is horizontal and snug but does not compress the skin. Now, relax, exhale, and note the circumference.

No complicated calculation is necessary. A waistline greater than thirty-five inches (for women) or forty inches (for men) is taken to mean you are carrying around an excess of abdominal fat. That increases the risk of diseases associated with obesity, which include diabetes, hypertension, heart disease and stroke, liver disease, certain cancers, irregular menstrual periods, sleep apnea, gallbladder disease, and the wear and tear of osteoarthritis.

If your BMI is greater than thirty *and* your waist circumference is above the female/male, thirty-five-inch/forty-inch threshold, lifestyle changes are in order. Consider the case of television newsman Tim Russert, who died suddenly of a heart attack in 2008. His cholesterol wasn't high, and his hypertension was controlled by medications, but he was overweight with a waist circumference in excess of forty inches. As his internist Dr. Michael A. Newman observed sadly, "If there's one number that's a predictor of mortality, it's waist circumference."

Take it as a warning.

Review the foods you have eaten in the last seventy-two hours. Next, answer these questions:

Q: *When choosing dairy foods, did you opt for low-fat milk and cheeses?*

Q: *Do the number of servings of fresh fruits and vegetables on the list outnumber the servings of processed foods?*

Q: *Do you avoid sugary or fatty snacks between meals?*

Q: *Do you eat more servings of fish, chicken, dried beans, eggs, and nuts than red meat?*

Q: *Do you drink more plain water than coffee, soda, and other beverages?*

Q: *Is your diet rich in fiber?*

If you answered "no" to some or all these questions, your diet is not helping you in your quest for longevity. Read on and rethink.

Strategy Eighteen: Review Your Eating Rituals

No single nutritional approach suits everyone. Our needs vary with age, sex, body type, activity level, the prescription drugs we take, and overall health status. Our culinary desires range widely, too, depending upon region, personal taste, and a multitude of other cultural, social, and economic factors. All of that makes a one-formula-fits-all solution for healthy eating impractical. At the same time, some of us find ourselves falling into rituals: We eat the same things over and over again, perhaps less out of choice than habit. Examining your eating routine may lead to healthier, more adventuresome, and perhaps more satisfying eating.

THE ASSIGNMENT. The best single tool at your disposal in considering what you eat is knowledge.

1. Before buying, ordering, selecting, or eating anything, recall that each bite of food and sip of liquid you swallow represents a choice; thus, a meal consists of many choices, a day's consumption of food many more.
2. Make it a habit to think—even for a nanosecond—about every eating decision you make, individually and collectively.

A FEW GUIDELINES. Informed dietary choices are essential to balancing your diet, controlling your weight, and enhancing your longevity. Consider these:

• *Variety is invaluable.* A healthy diet consists of a broad mix of foods. You should select nutrient-dense foods that are rich in vitamins and minerals. It should be a diverse mix, drawn mainly from these five food categories, namely grains; vegetables and fruits; low-fat milk and milk products; the meat and beans group; and the fats and oils (see *Eating Well for Long Life*, page 187). The foods in a sixth category—sweets and fatty deserts—are to be regarded as occasional treats, not staples, and should be consumed only in moderation.

• *Make menu selections with care.* In choosing foods at the store, remember that processing often robs them of essential vitamins and minerals, and too many simple sugary ingredients simply are not healthy. At restaurants, keep in mind that frying introduces excess fats.

• *Know that how much you eat is as important as what you eat.* We tend to need fewer calories with the passing years. As we age, we become less active than in younger years; in addition, our metabolism gradually slows (by age seventy-five, our basal metabolic rate, the pace at which our internal fires burn, drops by about 10 percent). That means we need less food to remain healthy and to maintain body weight. Just as we adapt our work and play habits to lessen the risks to our aging muscles and bones, our diets should evolve to reflect our changing needs.

- *Read ingredients lists.* Knowing precisely what is in a food product is vitally important. Prepackaged foods are required to list their ingredients in descending order of weight; the higher its name appears on the list, the greater amount of the ingredient is in the food. That's a good thing with whole grains, a bad thing with sugars and fats.

- *Learn the lingo.* Not everything in an ingredients list is what it may seem at first. All of the following are added sugars: corn syrup or sweetener, fruit juice concentrates, honey, molasses, brown or raw sugar, dextrose, fructose, glucose, lactose, maltose, or sucrose (and this is not a comprehensive list). When it comes to grains, "enriched" flour means some vital vitamins and minerals have been added; however, that enrichment is necessary because the processing has destroyed some of those same nutrients that originally were in the grain. That makes "whole" (that is, unprocessed) grains a preferred choice for half or more of your daily grain consumption.

- *Be educated about fats.* You have heard the argument: Too much fat can cause heart disease, especially saturated fats, and it is true. However, your body requires some fats to remain healthy, and some fats are healthier than others (see *Know Your Fats*, page 190).

- *Maintain a healthy weight.* Weight loss is, one way or another, about eating less. Often, however, a key element of a weight loss plan is to eat more of the right foods and less of the wrong ones. The best weight loss program for you—and the one that is less likely to result in a rebound weight gain—takes a slow and steady approach. Make small decreases in food and beverage calories. Eat smaller portions. Use a smaller plate. Resist the temptation to have seconds. Integrate other lifestyle changes—in particular regular physical activity.

- *Keep track of the total.* Whatever your health status but, in particular, if you are overweight, tracking your total caloric consumption can be valuable. For most average women, a total in the range of 1,600 calories per day is a good target; for men, 2,000 is regarded as a good baseline. It is not hard to make this calculation; it is a matter of keeping track of your consumption for a few days and then consulting widely available food charts (the United States Department of Agriculture publishes the comprehensive National Nutrient Database; check at your library or online at www.nal.usda.gov/fnic/foodcomp/Data/SR17/wtrank/sr17a208.pdf).

- *Have a plan in mind.* The best plans are not theoretical: They're practical, usable approaches that you can live with. The more you know, the more you think through your eating decisions, the better the odds you will eat a healthy diet.

antioxidants: an easy answer?

Back in high school biology class, I learned that the human body is made up of *cells.* My chemistry teacher taught me that the cells are composed of a variety of *molecules,* which consist of *atoms* linked by chemical *bonds.* I came to understand that when we eat, breathe, move, or do anything, the molecular makeup of our bodies changes as negatively charged particles in atoms (*electrons*) are shared with other atoms when chemical bonds are formed.

Free radicals. Back when I was in school, they didn't teach us about free radicals. Although most chemical bonds produce stable molecules with paired electrons spinning around them, the splitting of some bonds results in the release of free radicals, molecules that have spare electrons. Free radicals tend to recombine quickly, and do so by stealing an atom from a neighboring cell. A cascading chain of such reactions can result, sometimes creating a million or more free radicals.

In the world around us, free radicals cause paint to peel, pipes to leak, and food to spoil. In our bodies, free radicals are a normal by-product of metabolism, and some are produced by the body's immune system to fight viruses and bacteria. But other free radicals pose a danger to our health: Those produced by exposure to sunlight, radiation, stress, pollution, fumes, and chemicals can cause aging, disease, and death by damaging our cells, injuring our tissues, body proteins, hormones, even our genetic code. By reacting with cell membranes and our DNA, the free radicals can cause essential cells to perform inefficiently or even die.

Antioxidants. Nature has an answer to the challenges posed by the free radicals. Antioxidants are chemicals that neutralize free radicals by lending one of their own electrons to form new stable molecules; they effectively protect the body from free-radical damage. The fat-soluble vitamin E is an antioxidant, as is the water-soluble vitamin C. Vitamin E may help prevent heart disease (by protecting against the formation of plaque in the artery walls). Vitamin C has been found to interfere with free radical formation that can result from pollution and tobacco smoke; in studies, a high intake of this vitamin has been correlated with a lower incidence of oral cancer. The vitamin A precursor beta-carotene is also an antioxidant, as is glutathione (your body makes it from watermelon and asparagus) and lycopene (the red pigment in tomatoes).

Disease prevention. Fruits and vegetables are excellent sources of antioxidants and, as usual, your best strategy is to eat a balanced diet, emphasizing fresh fruit and vegetables. Five to eight servings a day will ensure an adequate intake of antioxidant nutrients. Foods rich in vitamin C include oranges, grapefruits, strawberries, green peppers, cabbage, spinach, broccoli, cantaloupe, kiwi, and kale. Vitamin E is found in such foods as nuts, seeds, apricots, vegetable and fish oils, whole grains, and fortified cereals. Beta-carotene occurs in liver, egg yolks, milk and butter, spinach, carrots, squash, broccoli, yams, tomatoes, cantaloupe, peaches, prunes, and grains. Glutathione is found in fish, walnuts, asparagus, and avocados. Artichokes have a flavonoid (an antioxidant) called silymarin.

As tempting as it may sound, a trip to the vitamin store for megadoses of antioxidants probably is not the answer. Large doses of antioxidants have uncertain effects, and researchers suspect that other chemicals found in fruits and vegetables (including flavonoids) may account for the cardiovascular effects of fruit and vegetable consumption.

Eating Well for Long Life

Since World War II, the United States government has issued dietary recommendations specifying how much of which nutrients constitute healthy nutrition. Canada and other countries also have published their own guidelines. Such standards have evolved over the years and, despite regular revisions, remain works in progress.

Many of the changes reflect new understandings of the role that nutrient deficiencies and excesses play in health and disease. Most recently the epidemic of obesity has been reflected in the various changes. The newest guidelines recommend a reduced intake of saturated and trans fats, as well as an increase in the consumption of various vitamins (B_{12} in people over fifty) and minerals (calcium).

I know there is no single perfect nutritional regime, whatever the claims of some diet book authors. Differences in age, sex, weight, height, physical activity level, health status, and other factors mean all of us need to tailor our diets to individuals needs. On the other hand, I can say with certainty that some essentials do apply across populations.

There are two basic ways to plan a diet. To oversimplify a bit, you can think like a cook or a chemist. The cook thinks about ingredients, and plans a meal by selecting an appealing mix of foods: meat and potatoes and vegetables, for example, or tofu, grains, and salad. The chemist looks at an array of foods in terms of what they contain, namely, nutrients, and thus the amount of protein, carbohydrates, vitamins, and minerals that a given combination of ingredients will provide. The thoughtful cook and the calculating chemist aim for the same goal—that is, a balanced, healthy diet—despite approaching the task from quite different angles.

In planning your diet, you will do best to think like both the cook and the chemist, but let's begin by looking at the raw foods that line your grocery store shelves. Our laboratory visit can come later.

FOOD CATEGORIES. You remember learning the basic food groups in your school days. The wisdom then was to eat a balanced diet consisting of meats, poultry, fish, dry beans and peas, eggs, and nuts; dairy products, such as milk, cheese, and yogurt; grains; and fruits and vegetables. While that has not changed radically, I prefer to think of sugars and oils apart from the other foods.

In planning your diet, then, you should set out to consume the following:

- Breads and other wheat products, pasta, cereals, rice, corn, and other grains: 6 to 11 servings daily
  - ❋ (1 serving = 1 slice of bread, 1 cup dry cereal, ½ cup cooked rice or pasta)
- Fruits (citrus, apples, banana, berries, etc.): 2 to 4 servings daily and vegetables (green and yellow vegetables, etc.): 3 to 5 servings daily
  - ❋ (1 serving = ½ cup)
- Milk and cheese: 2 to 3 servings daily
  - ❋ (1 cup milk or 1½ to 2 ounces cheese)
- Meat, poultry, fish, dry beans, eggs, and nuts: 2 to 3 servings daily
  - ❋ (total of 5½ to 6 ounces meat, poultry, fish, or equivalent from other sources such as eggs, beans, or nuts (1 ounce equivalents in such foods are 1 egg or ½ cup cooked dry beans or ½ ounce seeds or 1½ ounces nuts)
- Fats, oils, and sugars: Use sparingly
  - ❋ (1 to 2 tablespoons oil, 1 to 1½ teaspoons sugar per day)

THE NUTRIENT APPROACH. The underlying goal of eating is to provide your body with the proper quantities of fuel of the right sort for maximum health, full function, and body maintenance. Your body metabolizes what you eat to give you energy, to repair itself, and to operate its systems. This requires a mix of food substances.

Once again, think back to high school science. We learned about the calorie, the unit of measurement used by scientists to calculate the energy in food. Proteins, fats, and carbohydrates have relatively high caloric content. Other foods like fiber, vitamins, and minerals have little or none, but they make possible other bodily functions. Your body requires adequate amounts of all of these; the Food and Nutrition Board of the National Academy Institute of Medicine publishes recommended intakes (for the most recent recommendations, see the full chart at www.iom.edu/Object .File/Master/21/372/0.pdf).

Getting acquainted with the basics can be useful, but trying to plan a diet based on remaining within the recommended daily allowances for protein and carbohydrates while paying due regard to getting an adequate intake of selenium, biotin, riboflavin, and dozens of other elements would require more calculations, research, time, and patience than most of us are ready to invest. Such a process would hardly seem calculated to deliver the tastiest meals to the dinner table.

On the other hand, when eating prepared foods it is very useful to make reference to the Nutrition Facts printed on the label. Food packagers are required to specify how much fat, cholesterol, salt, carbohydrates, and protein are found in the food contained in each package, as well as what the amount cited represents of the recommended daily intake.

Here again, a certain amount of decoding is important. Be sure to check out the serving size: What may seem like an acceptable amount of fat in a serving may actually be very much more if the serving size is small and, as a result, you are likely to consume two or more servings. Potato chips are a classic case in point: If a serving size is 1 ounce, then the fat content is probably about 10 grams. If you eat an 8-ounce bag—which may at first may not seem like very much—you will have eaten roughly *twice* the recommended number of grams of fat that a normal adult should consume *in an entire day.* Always be watchful for *saturated fat* and *trans fats*, as well as for sugar and salt (sodium).

The single best way to improve your eating habits is to think before you eat *anything*, since every bite of food you take represents a choice. Is it on your plan? Is it a healthy food or is it on your not-recommended list? Ignorance is not bliss when it comes to consuming unhealthy foods; knowledge can give you the power to say no.

Another way to think about eating is in terms of portions. In general, smaller portions are the easiest way to cut down your intake; take a smaller portion of the well-marbled steak at dinner and double up on plain baked potato or steamed asparagus. You do not have to go hungry.

Be aware that prepared foods are more generous today than they used to be. The average bagel in today's marketplace is 150 percent larger than it was twenty years ago. Soft drink servings, hamburgers, muffins, cookies, and sandwiches have doubled and trebled in size. That 16-ounce mocha coffee the barista serves you today has seven or eight times the calories a cup of coffee with milk and sugar did in the diner of old.

As you think about making nutritional changes, picture yourself eating with other people: Breaking bread in concert with friends and family is nurturing in so many ways.

know your fats: friend and foe

Fats are not evil by definition. Yes, too much fat, particularly of the wrong sort, is demonstrably bad for you. But, as is so often true in matters of nutrition, the sensible application of a little moderation is appropriate.

Some dietary fat is essential for good health. Some fatty acids cannot be synthesized by the body and therefore must come from dietary sources. Within the body, these *essential fatty acids* (EFAs) are metabolized for a wide range of uses, including the absorption of vitamins A, D, E, and K and for the maintenance of cell membranes. Fats also play a role in the function of our hormones and immune system, taste good, and enhance digestion. In mechanical terms, body fats cushion our muscles, bones, and organs, and provide insulation. When our blood sugar is low, the body burns fat for needed energy.

That's the good news. The other side of the discussion involves the risks posed by excess fat consumption. The consumption of foods rich in animal fats has long been associated with the higher incidence of cancers, including breast and prostate, as well as cardiovascular disease.

Kinds of fats. The fats found in olive, sesame, canola, almond, flax, and fish oils contain *monounsaturated fats,* the healthiest category of fats. Much less desirable are the *polyunsaturated fats*, such as margarine and the oils of safflower, sunflower, and corn. They tend to be highly refined, and the spreadable hydrogenated fats contain large amounts of trans fats, which have been linked to heart disease and cancer. The third class of fat, *saturated fats*, also pose a significant health hazard. Consumption of saturated fats should be limited because these fats tend to elevate blood cholesterol and triglyceride levels, putting you at greater risk for stroke and heart attack. The saturated fats include butter, lard, palm, peanut, and coconut oils, as well as the fats found in eggs, cheese, beef, pork, chicken, and other meats. Fried foods in general tend to be high in saturated fats.

Fats in your diet. Although you need fat, you should consume no more than 10 percent of your daily caloric intake as saturated fats. Your total fat intake should be between 20 and 35 percent of your daily calories. Avoid foods high in saturated or trans fats.

A shopping suggestion. Much of the oil on grocery store shelves has been processed (distilled, extracted, refined, bleached, or defoamed) and the vegetables, seeds, or nuts from which the oils are derived may have been treated with pesticides and preservatives. Consequently, you may wish to invest in the more expensive organic, pressed olive or flaxseed oils. Purchase the ones in dark glass containers, which protect them from sunlight. The expense will be greater, but so will be the flavors.

Strategy Nineteen: Obey the Nutritional Ten Commandments

The following are ten recommendations for good nutrition—and good health. They can work for you.

THE ASSIGNMENT. My suggestion is as follows:

1. First, read and consider these ten advisories.
2. Next, examine your diet to figure out how you can obey these commandments and improve your dietary habits.

1. *Drink enough water.* Clean, fresh water quenches a thirst better than any other beverage. *Aim for 1½ to 2 quarts daily.*

2. *Eat less salt.* After age fifty, it is especially important to limit salt consumption. Use it sparingly in cooking and at the table; avoid prepared foods with high sodium content, which include breads, frozen pizza, canned soups, chips, and salad dressing. *Consume no more than 1,500 mg of sodium per day.*

3. *Eat more legumes and other leafy, dark green, and orange vegetables.* Legumes are foods that come in a pod, including most beans, peas, lentils, and soy. They're excellent sources of fiber, complex carbohydrates, protein, and minerals (experiment with tasty black beans, black-eyed peas, chickpeas, kidney beans, and lentils). *Have 2 to 2½ cups per day.*

4. *Eat less fat.* Many American consume fully half of their calories as fats; a healthier level would be between one-third and one-fifth of one's daily caloric consumption. In particular, avoid cholesterol-rich animal fats and trans fats, tipping the balance instead to sources of polyunsaturated and monounsaturated fatty acids like fish, nuts, and vegetable oils. *No more than 10 percent of your calories should be saturated fats.*

5. *Consume more fresh fruits.* They contain vitamins, minerals, fiber, and antioxidants galore. *Have 2 cups or more per day.*

6. *Emphasize whole grains.* Make sure you consume ample whole-grain products daily (at least half of the 6 ounces recommended daily amount of grains). In addition to familiar grains like wheat, corn, and oats, try other whole grains like millet and quinoa. The rest can come from enriched sources. *Eat 3 ounces or more each day.*

7. *Drink low-fat milk and milk products.* Whole milk contains about 4 percent fat; low-fat contains 1 or 2 percent. One cup milk or 1½ to

2 ounces cheese per serving. Consume 1 cup milk or 1½ to 2 ounces cheese per day.

8. *Beware added sugars.* Read the labels. Keep in mind your body requires no processed sugar. The complex carbohydrates you eat are broken down to keep your blood sugar levels balanced.

9. *Limit alcohol consumption.* Restrict your consumption of alcoholic beverages. Women and lighter men should consume no more than one drink a day and average-size and larger men less than two daily. If you have difficulty drinking in moderation, abstain from alcohol.

10. *Take a daily multivitamin.* After age sixty, it is good insurance.

alcohol: tonic or toxin?

Alcohol isn't truly a food—it has no nutritive value—but just as what you eat impacts your health, so does your consumption of alcohol.

Is it a tonic? Countless studies—more than a hundred in recent years—have been devoted to the impact of alcohol consumption on cardiovascular disease, and some have found that moderate drinking has some apparent health benefits. This research does not demonstrate the health-giving mechanism at the cellular level, since most of the studies look at trends in large populations, but people who tipple a little tend to live a little longer. Moderate wine drinkers may have a lesser risk of dementia; moderate alcohol consumption reduces the risk of infection with *Helicobacter pylori*, the bacterium that causes most stomach ulcers; women who drink conservatively have better bone density; and in retirement communities, moderate drinking is associated with better socialization and appetite.

Or is alcohol a toxin? On the negative side—and there most certainly is one—some of the same studies identified such hazards of excessive drinking as increased risk of heart disease, diabetes, bone demineralization (osteoporosis), social isolation, breast cancer, accidents (falls and incidents behind the wheel), and for chemical interactions that can lessen the desired effects of some medications and increase the potential toxicity of others.

How do we balance this equation? There are variables, of course, having to do with our personality, sex, physical size, health status, and many other factors. But if you are going to drink, you need to find the point of balance that is right for your health. Or you should not drink at all.

Drinking alcohol in moderation. Many studies suggest that, while a drink a day may not keep the doctor away, more than two quickly erases whatever benefit moderate alcohol consumption gains you. Other studies support a working assumption that, for maximum longevity, an average of one drink a day for men is probably ideal and up to two drinks a day is acceptable. For women, the ceiling should be perhaps half the men's average because their bodies metabolize alcohol more slowly, meaning the effects of the alcohol may be greater and longer lasting.

When is alcohol a health risk? For some people, there is no stopping at two: The best resolutions, lubricated by a little alcohol, suddenly disappear. If two drinks seem to lead inevitably to a third or even more drinks, abstinence may be the only solution. If you have chronic liver disease, poorly controlled hypertension, kidney disease, certain heart disorders, or you take medications that have adverse interactions with alcohol, you should avoid alcohol altogether.

Even in the absence of chronic disease, alcohol's effects change with the passing years. As we age, the body metabolizes alcohol more slowly than in earlier years. That means that, after having a drink, our blood alcohol rises more quickly and remains there longer. The increased sensitivity and decreased tolerance translates to a higher level of intoxication: The two drinks that relaxed you at forty-five may impair your judgment, make you unsteady on your feet, and cloud your thinking and memory at sixty-five.

To drink or not to drink. Look at your habits; if your alcohol consumption exceeds the recommended limits, rethink your rituals. This is a change you make for yourself, but you can learn and benefit from the guidance and goodwill of others. Controlling your alcohol consumption may be essential to your longevity.

Understanding the Organic

These days it is impossible to negotiate the aisles of a supermarket without encountering the term "organic." That is a word with multiple usages and, I would suggest, one worth thinking about for a moment.

To the chemist, organic identifies compounds containing carbon. To the biologist, it describes any material that is derived from living organisms. Given its implication of natural growth, the word has utility in the languages of computing, economics, and the law, but it is its agricultural usage that concerns us here.

In simpler times, all the plant and animal products produced by indigenous agriculture were organic. Then the farm was largely self-sufficient: The farmer cultivated plants and raised animals for food; an interdependence evolved. The plants grew in the soil and were harvested to feed humans and animals; in turn, the animals provided other foodstuffs for the humans as well as manure to replace nutrients in the soil. According to this model, everything was local, part of a sustainable life cycle that evolved over the millennia.

In the nineteenth century, advances in chemistry brought artificial fertilizers to the fields. Along with mechanization, the result was an increase in the scale of farming. The twentieth century saw the widespread introduction of pesticides, which reduce crop loss to insects, unwanted weeds, and certain microorganisms. Livestock began to be given growth hormones and antibiotics. The result of such advances was vastly increased yields and profits and the broad distribution of foods. The advent of chemicals meant the process was no longer organic.

There have been many and varied consequences of the shift to large-scale, chemically dependent farming. The emphasis on high-yield products has led to a reduction in biodiversity. The microbial activity of the soil has been interrupted, resulting in plants that depend upon the nutrients and other additives the farmer applies. Runoff from the fields results in pesticides in groundwater. And the meat, poultry, and dairy products grown by conventional means typically contain measurable amounts of pesticides, antibiotics, and sometimes hormones.

A debate continues to rage between advocates for conventional and organic farming. Organic farmers argue their more natural produce is safer and better tasting; the other side argues the risk of trace amounts of chemicals is small compared to the compelling need to maintain high production to feed a hungry world. Organic advocates claim their methods are less harmful to the environment; on the other hand, the produce that comes from conventional farms is usually more affordable.

Ultimately, the American consumer will decide the future of organics in American agriculture, but a decided taste for the organic has emerged in the marketplace. Organic products are far from dominant; yet organically grown fruit, vegetables, and meats are no longer merely a niche market serviced by specialty stores (more organic foods are now purchased in supermarkets, including national purveyors like Wal-Mart, than in smaller venues, suggesting a market shift is underway). Some organic farmers suffered during the economic downturn of 2008–2009, as consumers have opted for cheaper alternatives, but organic choices are here to stay.

The definition of organic was long open to interpretation, so the United States Department of Agriculture now issues and administers organic standards. USDA's National Organic Standards Board requires that foods labeled organic be produced without using most conventional pesticides, petroleum-based fertilizers, sewage sludge–based fertilizers, bioengineering, or ionizing radiation. Organic meat, poultry, eggs, and dairy products must come from animals that have been given no antibiotics or growth hormones. Farms that are certified organic are required to employ renewable resources and conserve soil and water. A government-approved certifier inspects the farms where the foods are grown to ensure the farmer meets USDA organic standards. Processors and handlers of organic food must also be certified.

The organic products at your grocery store offer you options; I suggest you experiment with organic alternatives to traditional choices if you have not already done so.

Strategy Twenty: Consume Needed Nutrients

In planning your menus, remember that the need for certain nutrients increases as we age. The body metabolizes foods differently in the aging years, and our cells have different needs.

THE ASSIGNMENT. Once again, the subject is choices; make sure that yours allow for the consumption of adequate supplies of essential nutrients.

THE FOODS. In choosing foods, select some that are rich in these nutrients:

- *Calcium.* Essential to strong and healthy bones at all ages, an ample supply of calcium can be found in milk, yogurt, and other dairy products (be sure to choose low-fat varieties). Other good sources are calcium-fortified breakfast foods and juices, dark leafy green vegetables, dried beans, almonds, and canned sardines or salmon.
- *Potassium.* Most Americans eat too little potassium, a mineral essential to regulating blood pressure and the body's fluid levels. Try to incorporate into your regular diet potatoes, tomatoes, spinach, bananas, oranges and orange juice, and soybeans, all of which are rich in potassium.
- *Magnesium.* Magnesium plays an important part in heart health, strong bones, and controlling blood pressure. One recent study suggests that increased magnesium intake may reduce the risk of type-2 diabetes in adults. Foods particularly rich in magnesium include bran cereals, cooked spinach, black beans, lima beans, Brazil nuts, roasted pumpkin seeds, and halibut.
- *Fiber.* Too many processed foods means less fiber; too little dietary

fiber can mean constipation (about 20 percent of people over sixty-five suffer from this discomfort regularly). Whole grains, fruits, and vegetable that are rich in fiber are also good sources of many vitamins, minerals, and other nutrients. Consumption of fiber may help you control how much you eat by making you feel satisfied more quickly. Fiber also helps reduce the absorption of cholesterol, leading to a reduced risk of heart disease and high blood pressure.

- *Vitamin A.* Research has found a reduced risk of heart disease for people who consume diets high in carotenoids. One carotenoid is the beta-carotene of vitamin A, the orange pigments in produce. Good sources of vitamin A include bright orange vegetables like carrots, sweet potatoes, pumpkin, tomatoes and tomato products, red sweet pepper, leafy greens (such as spinach, collards, turnip greens, kale, beet and mustard greens, and lettuce), and orange fruits (mango, cantaloupe, apricots, and red or pink grapefruit).

- *Vitamin C.* This vitamin has been credited with all sorts of curative powers; some are exaggerated, but certainly vitamin C (also known as ascorbic acid) is essential to healthy blood and brain function, among many other bodily duties. Fruits and vegetables are the primary sources, especially citrus fruits and juices, kiwis, strawberries, guava, papaya, cantaloupe, broccoli, peppers, tomatoes, cabbage (especially Chinese cabbage), Brussels sprouts, and potatoes, as well as leafy greens such as romaine lettuce, turnip greens, and spinach.

- *Vitamin D.* This nutrient has garnered more than a little attention in recent years for its role in healthy bones (its presence allows the body to use calcium properly). It also plays essential roles in managing blood pressure, insulin balance, and the body's immune system. Good sources of vitamin D are fortified dairy products, eggs (yolks in particular), liver, and saltwater fish. Exposure to the sun is important, too, as it enables your body to make vitamin D (ten to fifteen minutes three times per week is sufficient).

- *Vitamin E* actually describes a family of eight antioxidants (see *Antioxidants: An Easy Answer?* on page 185), the principal one being alpha-tocopherol. Good sources include nuts (almonds, hazelnuts, peanuts and peanut butter), oils (olive, soybean, corn, canola, safflower, and sunflower), avocados, spinach, and carrots.
- *Vitamin supplements.* You may also wish to consider taking vitamin and mineral supplements in case dietary sources do not provide you with adequate supplies of necessary nutrients (see *Adam's Apothecary*, page 206).

dental health

We tend to take our teeth for granted—until, that is, they begin to hurt or even fall from our mouths. As a young man, George Washington cracked walnuts with his; as he aged, his once healthy bite deteriorated, eventually leaving him toothless and in need of dentures (made not of wood but hippopotamus ivory and human teeth). Modern dentistry has come a very long way since the Founding Fathers' era, but your attention to oral health is essential.

Tooth enamel is the hardest substance found in the human body, but the aging process exacts a toll on the teeth. The enamel erodes with age; the blood supply to the roots and tooth pulp decreases, as does the flow of saliva. Cavities can occur at any age; gum problems can result in inflammation called periodontal disease or gingivitis. If left untreated, the gums will swell and bleed and, eventually, like General Washington's, your teeth may fall out.

See your dentist regularly. All of which is an argument for regular checkups and cleaning; six-month intervals make sense, unless you have issues that require extra attention. Your dentist will also conduct an examination for oral cancers, which are more likely in the aging years, and to help ensure that your dentures or other appliances fit and function properly.

Brush twice daily. A thorough brushing in the morning and night of all the teeth surfaces is essential.

Use anti-sensitivity toothpaste. Some minor tooth discomfort, such as sensitivity to hot and cold, can be alleviated by the use of specially formulated but generally available toothpastes. If, however, the discomfort persists, be sure to discuss the symptoms with your dentist to be certain it is not a cavity, cracked tooth, or other dental problem requiring treatment.

Floss daily. Floss once a day in order to remove food particles and other matter the toothbrush cannot reach or dislodge.

Avoid tobacco and minimize alcohol. Your oral health can be compromised by tobacco and alcohol.

Seek solutions to other complaints. If you experience dry mouth, a common side effect of many medications, talk to your physician and your dentist about options. If you have lost teeth or some have loosened, there are dental solutions, ranging from crowns and bridges to permanent implants.

Moderating Consumption

At sixty-one, Wendy went to see her physician for a checkup. She was in perfect health, she thought, so she felt only a little guilty at having let four years elapse since her last checkup. Her doctor remarked on it. "An annual visit is free, you know, with your health insurance." Properly chastised, she promised to do better in the future.

The doctor did indeed pronounce her health very good—as far he could tell. He did say he wanted to see the results of her blood work before making any final pronouncements, but Wendy was surprised when the nurse called with word that her cholesterol was elevated.

"Really?" she asked.

"It's 255," she was told.

For a moment, Wendy worried about this. She had gone through meno-pause seven years earlier and, she remembered, lots of women are at greater risk of heart disease without the protective effects of estrogen. She took that as the explanation, since in other ways her life had not changed really at all for many years.

The nurse had said something else, too, that Wendy had to think about. "The doctor wants to see you in sixty days. You should try to get your number down, because he's probably thinking about a cholesterol-reducing drug."

That idea worried Wendy more than the lab results. Not that she doubted the cholesterol–heart disease connection, which seemed probable enough to her. But she had seen her mother in her last years taking all kinds of drugs. The meds, it seemed to Wendy, had taken as much of a toll on her health as her various ailments had.

Always a task-oriented person, Wendy decided to do as she had been advised. She eliminated cookies and brownies and other sweets from her diet. She knew they were a big part of the problem. She ate oatmeal al-most every morning (fortunately, it was winter). She cooked at home more, where she could control the ingredients. Pizza was out. She ate more fish and chicken; when red meat was on offer, she limited herself to small portions. No butter added. Ever. Ice cream was for other people. Her hus-band, an excellent baker, was told to put away his baking pans for a while. She made every dietary change she could think of to bring down her fat consumption.

Another nurse called to tell her of an appointment for a blood test ("He wants the results before he sees you," she advised). Wendy arrived at the doctor's offer more than ready to find out how she had done on the test.

The doctor looked at her squarely. "I have to save that little speech I was going to give you," he said, his face breaking into a smile. "You dropped your cholesterol fifty-five points in sixty days. I'm impressed."

Wendy couldn't help but smile back. The lesson? You can take control of your diet—and your health.

Strategy Twenty-one:
Make Healthy Food Choices

Weight loss, cholesterol reduction, and blood-sugar management: Those are tasks that can be accomplished by strategic and disciplined dietary change. The process can be greatly enhanced by an accompanying program of regular physical activity (see *Prescription VI: Live the Active Life*, page 138), but the fuel we put into the engine has an all-important impact.

THE ASSIGNMENT. Healthy eating involves limiting your intake of foods high in fats and sugars, but it does not mean you should eat less of everything. Think *dos* and *don'ts* as you dine.

NUTRITIONAL APPROACHES. Here are some suggestions for managing your diet:

- *Eat a little less.* Portion control is essential: Increase the foods high in fiber, and take more modest servings of those high in fat. Avoid seconds. Try to stop eating before you are full. Eat more slowly (that way the *I'm-getting-full* message has a better chance of reaching your brain before you overeat).
- *Eat smaller meals.* You might find it remarkable how using a smaller plate helps you eat less.
- *Eat your larger meals earlier.* Much research suggests that proteins and fats eaten at breakfast are more likely to be burned during the day, delivering you energy you need rather than getting stored in your body.
- *Think colors.* Food is about more than taste (and the related sense of smell). Visual appeal is important, too, so as you think about vegetables, incorporate colors: red peppers, yellow squash, green

beans, deep red beets, white potatoes, yellow yams, black mushrooms. When it comes to fruits, the choices are also varied. Melons alone are red, green, and orange; apples red and green and yellow; bananas yellow (skin) and white (flesh).

- *An apple a day?* Apple, plums, lemons, cranberries, and grapefruit contain pectin, which has been shown to help reduce cholesterol in the blood. Fresh fruit is health-giving in other ways, too, as a source of fiber (good for digestive regularity).

- *Brown rice is better rice.* White rice is brown rice with the hull removed. When the bran coating is stripped off, so are various B vitamins and vitamin E. Again, brown rice is a good source of fiber.

- *Whole grains are wholesome.* This is one message that cannot be repeated too many times: Eat whole grains. They are richer in dietary fiber, calcium, magnesium, and potassium than are processed and enriched grains. Oats, for example, as with rice, lose the outer coating (the oat bran) in processing, which has health-giving properties. Bran fibers bind to various substances, helping to speed the excretion of cholesterol and certain toxic minerals. Other whole grains are barley, whole wheat, shredded wheat, brown rice, wild rice, barley, popcorn, buckwheat, bulgur, whole rye, amaranth, and quinoa.

- *Nitrite-free hot dogs . . . if you must.* Hot dogs are not exactly a health food, but those with nitrates (food preservatives used to prevent botulism in cured meats including hot dogs) are definitely not on the recommended list. Nitrites combine with dietary amines to form known carcinogens called nitrosamines. Read the label before your next purchase of hot dogs; nitrite-free hot dogs are safe.

- *Exploit the potato.* An amazing food is the potato. It is rich in potassium, vitamin C, and fiber. A whole potato, with skin, constitutes only about 125 calories when eaten plain. Beware high-fat toppings like gravy, butter, and sour cream; try yogurt, salsa, beans, cucumbers, onions, low-fat cheeses, cottage cheese, fruits, or lean meats. The sweet potato may be even healthier than the plain potato, with even more nutrients—*and* more flavor.

- *Go low-salt.* The body needs salt, but approximately 1 teaspoon daily is enough for most people, and too much for those with hypertension. Perhaps three-quarters of the salt we eat is not added in cooking or at the table but in processing, so read food labels carefully. Studies have found that a high level of salt consumption is a risk factor for hypertension; for cancers of the esophagus, stomach, and bladder; and for osteoporosis. For those who have hypertension, it is definitely not on the table. You might try sea salt rather than the bland, refined table salt. Sea salt has dozens of trace minerals the body needs.

- *Beware of food additives.* Lots of substances are used to preserve foods—but sometimes with unwanted consequences. In sensitive individuals, for example, MSG (monosodium glutamate) can trigger headaches. Sulfites are chemicals used in food processing to inhibit discoloration (browning) of certain foods (such as shrimp and potatoes), as well as in the manufacture of wine, beer, and a wide variety of medications. In sensitive individuals, sulfites can trigger wheezing and even full-blown asthmatic reactions.

- *Eat like a hunter-gatherer.* Nuts, seeds, and berries contain a range of healthful nutrients. Nuts and seeds contain arginine, a protein that keeps your arteries flexible, and the skins of cranberries and blueberries are high in antioxidants. Berries tend to be small in size, intense in flavor, and rich in vitamins. Nuts have lots of fiber, too.

- *Eat your spinach.* It may not make you the strong man as it did Popeye, but spinach is something of a wonder food: low in calories, high in fiber, vitamins, minerals, and antioxidants, meaning it may well help protect you against cancer and heart disease. Kale and collard greens are other leafy green vegetables that are widely available.

- *Wash before eating.* Thoroughly rinse fresh food items to remove the residue of pesticides and fungicides.
- *Flavor your foods.* If you are embarking on a weight-reduction plan, try adding interest to your diet. Flavor your food with herbs and spices, modest amounts of vinegar, and garlic and ginger. For centuries ginger has been used as an herbal remedy, but more recently claims have been made for its anticancer properties (it contains the antioxidant geraniol) and as an anti-inflammatory. Garlic is another flavoring agent with a difference. The presence of an organic compound called allicin may make garlic useful in preventing atherosclerosis and hypertension. It may also boost the immune system. Spices can aid digestion, so moderate amounts of cooking spices such as anise, basil, bay leaf, cardamom, dill, fennel, ginger, and mustard may have a beneficial impact on the way your gastrointestinal tract processes what you eat. Their tastes and smells can add appeal to meals that are low in fat.
- *Nuts are your friends.* A large Harvard study determined that participants in a group who consumed olive oil, almonds, and other nuts (which contain monounsaturated fats) while on a low-fat diet lost as much weight as those who were on a low-calorie, low-fat diet. Further, researchers found that six months later, the nut eaters had kept the weight off while the other dieters were gaining it back.
- *Emphasize fish.* In general, fish is lower in fat than meat. In addition, the presence of omega-3 fatty acids may have a range of protective effects, including a reduction in the risk of coronary artery disease. (That said, most fish and shellfish also contain traces of mercury, so moderation should be the rule: I recommend no more than two meals a week with 6-ounce servings of fish. Opt for shrimp, canned light tuna, salmon, pollack, and catfish, since shark,

swordfish, king mackerel, white or albacore tuna, and tilefish should be consumed only rarely because they have measurably higher levels of mercury.)

adam's apothecary

Food sources are the best way to get the vitamins, microminerals, and trace minerals (together called micronutrients) that your body needs. However, the aging process can mean that the body absorbs dietary sources less efficiently. Deficiencies of vitamin B_{12} (which can lead to anemia) and vitamin D (essential to the absorption of calcium into the bones) thus become more likely.

As the name implies, *supplements* should be secondary to a healthy diet consisting of as many fresh and varied foods as possible. A daily multivitamin pill simply is not a substitute for a good diet.

The daily multivitamin. After age sixty, taking certain dietary supplements on a daily basis may be a good strategy. A daily multivitamin tablet is a modest insurance policy (tablets generally are cheaper than capsules or liquids). Most multivitamins contain a mix of essential vitamins and minerals, including vitamins A, C, D, E, and a mix of B vitamins (including B_6 and B_{12}), as well as such minerals as calcium, magnesium, and iron. Read the label for quantity: A megadose is not required, but a multivitamin that provides 100 percent of the Recommended Daily Value for the nutrients is best. You may also find preparations formulated especially for older people, which will have lesser amounts of iron and more calcium and B vitamins. Products that claim to be all-natural, time-release, and easier to absorb (chelated) are usually more expensive but not necessarily better.

For some people, added supplements of certain individual vitamins and minerals are appropriate.

Calcium. This mineral is the bone builder; too little of it stored in your bones means increased risk of the bone demineralization of osteoporosis. Much attention has been devoted to calcium deficiencies for women, but after age fifty both men and women should be sure to consume 1,200 mg of calcium daily. You may wish to take a calcium supplement to be sure. Calcium supplementation is most effective when taken more than once a day in amounts less than 500 mg per dose.

Vitamin B_{12}. The latest USDA nutritional guidelines recommend that, in order to ensure people over fifty get enough of this key vitamin, they should eat cereal fortified with vitamin B_{12} or take a B_{12} supplement. While many meats (among them calf's liver, beef, and lamb) are high in vitamin B_{12}, the aging body tends to absorb vitamin B_{12} from dietary sources less efficiently.

Vitamin D. Older adults, especially those who get little exposure to sun, may have vitamin D deficiencies. Most basic one-a-day vitamin supplements should provide sufficient vitamin D.

Magnesium. The typical daily vitamin and mineral supplement contains 50 to 100 mg. Be aware, however, that too much magnesium is not healthful; your daily intake should not exceed 350 mg.

Talk to your physician. Discuss the appropriateness of vitamin or mineral supplements beyond a one-a-day vitamin with your doctor before you begin taking them. Some of them interact with prescription drugs or may be inappropriate if you have certain health issues. Your physician may have recommendations about substitute or additional supplements.

the abcs of beverages

We could no more survive without precious water than we could without food. Fortunately, our sources of liquid refreshment are plentiful; unfortunately, not every available liquid is good for us.

More. One of the oddities of the aging process is that our bodies tend to send us fewer *I-am-thirsty* messages as we age. In older people, the kidneys also function less efficiently in conserving water; taken together, that can put us at risk of dehydration. Since the body needs water to dissolve waste products, facilitate excretion, and lubricate itself in a hundred different ways, the lesson is clear: *Drink sufficient water every day.* For the average person, that means a minimum of 1½ to 2 quarts of water.

Less. Lots of people drink an excess of carbonated beverages. The phosphoric acid in such drinks increases your risk of osteoporosis by reducing bone density. Many Americans consume more than 100 pounds of sugar a year, and not a little of it comes from sweetened beverages. Sugary, carbonated drinks typically contain the equivalent of ten teaspoons of sugar. Plain water is the healthier choice.

Alcoholic beverages. Numerous studies suggest that moderate alcohol consumption reduces the risks of coronary heart disease. However, that benefit quickly disappears when alcohol is consumed immoderately, and there is evidence that binge drinking (defined as five or more drinks) damages the heart. Women and lighter weight men should limit consumption of alcoholic beverages to no more than one drink a day, average and heavier men to two or less. (See also *Alcohol: Tonic or Toxin?* on page 193.)

Caffeinated beverages. Like soda, caffeine can reduce bone mass. The compounds in coffee have many effects on the body, one of which is to stimulate the adrenal glands to produce stress hormones. Caffeine also raises blood pressure, so limiting caffeine-containing beverages is a good strategy for certain individuals, among them people with hypertension. For people in good overall health who enjoy coffee and cola drinks, moderation should rule.

The Longevity Diet?

Is there such a thing? The answer to that difficult question is not clear, as scientists continue to tease ambiguous results from long-term investigations. New findings are being published regularly, but the data is subject to interpretation.

Consider the results of a study published in July 2009 in *Science* magazine under the title "Caloric Restriction Delays Disease Onset and Mortality in Monkeys." The much anticipated report, based on an ongoing, twenty-year-long study of rhesus monkeys, looked at the surviving monkeys, all of which were at least twenty-seven years old, the rhesus equivalent of old age. The study reported that just five of the original thirty-eight calorie-restricted monkeys had died from age-related causes, compared to fourteen of thirty-eight in the control group. That no doubt led to the headlines that soon appeared in the media, which claimed unambiguously that calorie-counting monkeys live longer.

As usual, the truth is more complicated, since other scientists who examined the data quickly pointed out that when monkeys who died of causes apparently unrelated to aging were added back into the statistics (the authors of the study had omitted them), life span was not significantly extended.

In short, then, we have yet to be presented with incontrovertible proof of the existence of a "longevity diet." On the other hand, monkeys in studies of calorie restriction (CR) have maintained a lower body temperature, had lower levels of insulin in their bloodstreams, and a slower onset of a variety of age-related diseases, including cancer, diabetes, heart disease, brain atrophy, and lean muscle loss. Such results suggest that, indeed, this avenue of investigations holds great promise.

All of which raises the big question: *So how about people?*

The premise of CR is that a diet that consists of 30 or 40 percent fewer calories than average will result in greater longevity. Lab mice on such CR diets do live longer than control mice who eat a more usual diet, but people don't live in labs, and we tend to have difficulty with the severe limitations on consumption that the regimen of a CR diet demands; to many, the necessary discipline resembles deprivation. But people who do manage to radically restrict caloric intake tend to have lower body mass, meaning they are slimmer. Some of them live long lives but, again, there is no certainty that eating a great deal less will result in a significantly longer life.

Solid findings do indicate a relationship between long-term calorie restriction and a reduced incidence of atherosclerosis. It has also been observed that people on CR diets exhibit a slower decline of certain heart functions that come with aging. As with the rhesus monkey, most individuals who consume a diet that has 30 to 40 percent fewer calories than average have lower levels of blood pressure, blood sugar, and triglycerides, reducing the risks of hypertension and diabetes as well as heart disease.

Bottom line? Good research being done by CR investigators may yet

YOUR FOUR STRATEGIES TO EATING WELL FOR LONGEVITY

Selecting healthy foods to enhance your health isn't always easy—but it is essential.

Strategy Eighteen: Review Your Eating Rituals

Think about your nutritional habits. Some changes may be in order; see page 182.

Strategy Nineteen: Obey the Nutritional Ten Commandments

Good sensible advice for wise nutrition: see page 191.

Strategy Twenty: Consume Needed Nutrients

As you age, certain nutrients become more important; for a list, see page 197.

Strategy Twenty-one: Make Healthy Food Choices

Be vigilant: Everything you put in your mouth may have a health impact; see page 202.

The goal is to balance the need to eat a healthy diet with the desire to eat with relish and pleasure.

demonstrate a cause-and-effect relationship between radically moderated calorie consumption and longevity, but for all the encouraging findings, much work remains to be done before I will be comfortable will the notion of a longevity diet. Yet even in absence of proof that eating less will help you live longer, it does seem reasonable to conclude that people who moderate their consumption of calories will increase their odds of living better, healthier lives.

PRESCRIPTION VIII

PRACTICE PREVENTION

❖

THE PREFERRED TERM THESE DAYS IS "PRIMARY CARE PHYSICIAN," but many of us still like to think of our doctor in more personal terms. We want to see someone more human than is implied by an insurance company acronym like HCP (health care provider). In truth, if we have to reveal our bodies and our secrets, most of us want a physician with whom we feel comfortable, someone sensitive to our anxieties.

Having the feeling that we are in good hands can be reassuring, but it is also important to recognize that the old doctor-patient model has been transformed. The one-stop shopping of the old days is largely gone; the doctor who asked a few questions, examined whatever it was that hurt, looked thoughtful, and then pronounced his diagnosis while writing a prescription has been replaced by the "gate-keeper." The typical physician today still gives good guidance for usual health and illness issues, but he or she is much quicker to order diagnostic tests or to refer us to other doctors, to specialists, when our problems go beyond the basic.

One thing that hasn't changed: To help ensure good long-term health and longevity, getting regular health care is important. You need a doctor, and you need to see him or her at regular intervals (at least annually). Having a doctor who knows you is invaluable not only when you are sick; a thorough medical examination is necessary for him or her to obtain a thorough understanding of your health status. Prevention is one of the keys to longevity; the three-decade dividend exists in large measure because of advances in care and prevention of lifestyle diseases.

Your doctor will wish to examine you head to toe. Today it is quite standard to take a sample of your blood in order that a lab can conduct a comprehensive analysis. Your blood pressure will be measured. An electrocardiogram (EKG) is also appropriate so your doc will have on hand a baseline record for comparison later if you should complain of chest pains or exhibit other symptoms of a cardiac event. The doctor will record a detailed medical history, asking not only what ailments you have or have had but about your parents and siblings. Tell him what medications you take; do not omit the alternative, over-the-counter medicaments you take, including vitamin, mineral, and herbal supplements. Your doctor will ask whether your immunizations are updated (see page 222).

Strategy Twenty-two: Master the Medical Tests

Modern medicine is putting a new emphasis on prevention, and screening tests are essential to that effort. These are the lab tests, scans, and other examinations used to identify undiagnosed health problems; when conducting a physical exam, your physician will probably order a mix of standard assessments. These may involve lab analyses, scans, and other evaluations.

THE ASSIGNMENT. As a consumer, as well as a patient, you need to have a basic understanding of each of the tests and what they mean. Some ailments—the classic example is hypertension—have no obvious symptoms in day-to-day life. The early diagnosis of certain cancers substantially increases the chance of a cure, while some chronic diseases can be prevented or, at least, minimized if early warning signs are recognized and steps taken to alter unhealthy behaviors or treat the early symptoms. In short, identifying health problems in people with no obvious symptoms allows for early treatment and longer, healthier lives.

On the other hand—and there is another side to the discussion—screening tests can produce false positives or false negatives (the former means the test indicates you have a disease that you do not have, while the latter occurs when a test fails to identify an existing disease). Some screening tests pose health risks: For example, a very small percentage of colonoscopies (in which a flexible tube is inserted into the rectum in order to capture images of the tissue) result in perforation of the bowel. These considerations make it all the more important that you understand the procedure, the risks, how the test results are to be interpreted, and what are the probable outcomes. Let your physician be your guide, but collecting other information from authoritative sources will give you a deeper perspective.

THE TESTS. Among the most common and essential are these:

- *Cholesterol screening.* A general physical examination includes the drawing of blood, usually after a twelve-hour fast. Laboratory instruments will then be used to determine the levels of fatty substances (lipids) in the blood, a key risk factor (when the cholesterol reading is high) for coronary artery disease. If you are found to have elevated blood cholesterol (especially the "bad" cholesterol,

LDL, or low-density lipoprotein), your doctor will likely talk to you about strategies for lowering blood fats through diet, exercise, and possibly medications (see *Heart and Vascular Disease*, page 244). *Frequency:* At least every five years, more often if blood lipids are elevated.

- *Fasting blood glucose.* This test needs to be done regularly to determine the amount of sugar (glucose) in your blood, since excess glucose in the blood is an early indicator of diabetes. Again, lifestyle changes or medications can control blood sugar to avoid the many complications of diabetes. (See *Diabetes in the Aging Years*, page 234.) *Frequency:* At least every three years, more often if glucose levels are elevated or there is a family history of diabetes.

- *Blood pressure.* Hypertension is easy to diagnose by a simple blood pressure test administered in the doctor's office (or just about anywhere, including grocery stores using a sphygmomanometer—that's the proper name for the cuff-and-gauge device your doctor wraps around your upper arm at checkup time. Without periodic blood pressure checks, hypertension is virtually undetectable, and puts you at risk for a number of serious disorders. (See *Managing Your Blood Pressure*, page 246.)

- *Colorectal screening.* Cancers of the colon and rectum can be identified early through a combination of a doctor's rectal exam, a lab test to determine whether there is hidden (occult) blood in the stool, and periodic colonoscopy to look for precancerous growths called discharge polyps. (See *Cancer Prevention*, page 236.) *Frequency:* Your doctor will likely perform a rectal exam during your regular physical. Depending upon other factors, including family history, it may be appropriate to perform more sophisticated tests at one-, three-, five-, or ten-year intervals.

- *Eye exam.* An ophthalmologist or optometrist should periodically examine your eyes for cataracts, glaucoma, and age-related macular degeneration, as well as vision loss. (See *Seeing and Hearing*, page 216.) *Frequency:* Every year or two, more often if you wear glasses or have an eye disorder.

- *Dental checkup.* Dental exams remain important throughout life, and your dentist will examine not only your teeth but the gums, soft tissues, tongue, and lips. (See *Dental Health,* page 199.) *Frequency:* At least once a year.

FOR WOMEN: A number of screening tests apply primarily to women. They include:

- *Breast exam.* Women should examine their breasts once a month for lumps, puckering, or other changes. Periodically your doctor should perform a clinical breast exam. *Frequency:* At least annually.
- *Mammography.* The mammogram is an X-ray photograph of the breast. A valuable screening tool in identifying abnormalities in the tissue, mammography studies indicate that regular mammograms lower a woman's risk of dying from breast cancer by one third. After much debate, the clear consensus is that women over fifty should have annual mammograms. The use of hormone replacement therapy increases the risk of breast cancer, so if you used HRT, be sure to stick to an annual schedule of mammograms. *Frequency:* Annually.
- *Pap smear.* The Papanicolaou test should be a ritual part of a younger woman's annual gynecological checkup (it is invaluable in the early detection of cervical cancer). After age sixty-five, annual tests may no longer be necessary if you have had a sequence of normal tests.
- *Bone density test.* This X-ray scan of the lower back can detect the loss of bone mass that leads to osteoporosis, more prevalent in women. *Frequency:* A baseline exam should be done soon after menopause. Discuss follow-up tests with your physician, as the

need will vary with the original finding, family history, and other factors.

- The *prostate-specific antigen* (PSA), which measures levels of PSA, can detect prostate cancer or other conditions. *Frequency:* Annually.

Seeing and Hearing

We tend to take our ability to see and hear for granted, but if those senses begin to fade, the effect on quality of life can be great. We rely on both sight and sound for mobility, safety, communication, and a thousand everyday tasks. Treating your eyes and ears with appropriate care in the aging years is a healthy strategy.

HEARING LOSS. A hearing deficit can make social exchanges more difficult, and feelings of uncertainty, frustration, and depression can result. In practical terms, employment and economic opportunities may be lost. Progressive hearing loss can result in isolation and loss of productive engagement in life.

Damage to the ear can have a profound effect on balance and spatial perception, too, resulting in difficulties walking and standing, vertigo, and even nausea. Hearing loss is a safety issue. Not being able to hear such warning noises as honking horns, machinery, or other cues puts the person with a hearing deficit at greater risk for everyday accidents.

The cause of hearing loss may be disease, the aging process, or genetic predisposition, but often deafness results from exposure to excessive noise. Improper ear care, exposure to certain harmful chemicals, and some medications can have an impact on your ability to hear, too.

There are four common types of preventable hearing loss and illness.

- *Noise-induced hearing loss.* Exposure to excessive noise accounts for roughly one in four cases of hearing loss. Noise-induced hearing loss (NIHL) tends to develop over a long period. Since it is painless, it often goes undetected before significant damage has occurred. Although it is usually irreversible, it is the easiest form of hearing loss to prevent.
- *Swimmer's ear.* External otitis, as it is also known, is an infection of the outer ear, which consists of the ear canal and eardrum. It usually occurs when bacteria develops in water caught the ear. Symptoms include outer ear pain and a feeling that the ear is clogged.
- *Glue ear.* Middle-ear otitis, also known as "glue ear," is caused by bacteria or viruses, which lead to the accumulation of pus or mucus behind the eardrum in the vicinity of the ear bones. The symptoms may be severe earache, feelings of fullness or pressure, hearing loss, difficulty swallowing, or fever. If left untreated, ear infections can lead to permanent hearing loss, but are much more common in children than adults.
- *Airplane ear.* Barotitis media or barotrauma, as it is also known, occurs when the ear's inner air pressure is out of sync with the surrounding environment; as the name suggests, this commonly occurs during rapid changes in altitude in an aircraft. Symptoms include a feeling of fullness in the ear, hearing loss, ear pain, dizziness, a ringing in the ears (tinnitus), vertigo, and even bleeding from the ear. Often simple strategies like yawning, swallowing, or chewing gum can prevent or correct the difference in air pressure and resolves airplane ear symptoms. However, a severe case of airplane ear may need to be treated by a doctor.
- The single best means of maintaining healthy hearing is to avoid exposure to loud noises, especially those that are intense, sustained, and near at hand.

When people describe a sound as "too loud," most often they are referring to the *intensity* of the sound. High-intensity sound damages hearing and balance, as it destroys the hair cells in the inner ear. Once destroyed, these hairs cannot be replaced. As a rule of thumb, if you need to raise your voice in order to be able to communicate with someone an arm's length away, you are being exposed to sound levels that are too intense and therefore damaging.

Sound *duration* is also a potential cause of hearing loss. Studies have found that prolonged exposure to not-quite-so-loud sounds (a busy road, a lawn mower, or a motorcycle engine, for example) can damage your hearing. Working an eight-hour shift in a loud restaurant, taking a two-hour motorcycle ride, or mowing a lawn for most of an afternoon all can produce hearing loss.

Sound *distance* is another factor. Thus, headphones are more likely to overpower your ears than speakers; the closer you are to the sound source, the more damage you may do to your ears.

- *Reduce the noise around you.* Avoid settings where the noise is overwhelming. In environments you can control, take measures to reduce the noise; an added result will be a reduction in stress and anxiety levels. Use mufflers on air intakes and exhausts; use sound-absorbent materials.
- *Wear ear protection.* If you are routinely exposed to loud noise, wear ear protection. Both earplugs (small inserts that fit into the outer ear) and ear muffs (which fit over the entire outer ear) can reduce noise levels. Make sure the devices fit properly, as poorly fitted earplugs offer little protection.
- *Consult your physician.* If you experience severe earache, feelings of fullness or pressure, difficulty swallowing, fever, sudden hearing loss, dizziness, a ringing in the ears (tinnitus), vertigo, or bleeding from the ear, see your doctor. You should have your hearing checked at two-year intervals, more often if you have hearing loss.
- *Hearing aids.* If you have sustained permanent hearing loss, the chances are still good that there is a hearing aid that can help you hear better. These devices—they are essentially miniature sound systems consisting of a microphone, amplifier, speaker, and a battery—collect sounds from

your environment, amplify them, and deliver them directly to your ear. The designs vary. Some are entirely in the ear canal, some are in the ear, and some are behind it. The prices range greatly, too, from hundreds to thousands of dollars.

Consult your physician for a referral to an audiologist to help you make the right choice. Keep in mind that your hearing loss represents a great deal more than missing a few sentences in conversation. Your ability to communicate with those you love, with passersby on the street, with coworkers and friends is compromised if you have a hearing loss. Being unable to hear environmental cues is a safety issue, too. And do not allow your vanity to get it in the way ("Oh, my, I'd look like a geezer!"). Most people will not notice; and if you are forever asking people to repeat themselves, that's probably worse. Being able to play a full part in the transactions going on around you is important to your quality of life.

VISION LOSS. We use our eyes to read books and faces. We look both ways before we cross the street. Our vision enables us to appreciate color, perspective, and pattern in our world, to look at our watches, search the Internet, drive, and watch the sunset. Most of us could not imagine living our lives without sight. It is such a basic function for most of us that we take it for granted, do little to maintain it, and simply resign ourselves to age-related vision loss.

Yet much blindness in the world—perhaps 80 percent of cases of those with cataracts, trachoma, glaucoma, diabetic retinopathy, and vision loss due to accidents—could be avoided with proper prevention and treatment. Recent studies suggest that, even in the Western world where proper eye care is generally available, the risk of age-related macular degeneration could be significantly reduced.

Appropriate precautions can preserve vision and, in many cases, stave off further vision problems for those who have already experienced vision loss.

- *Age-related macular degeneration.* AMD is the leading cause of blindness in the Western world. An estimated eight million persons worldwide are blind or severely visually impaired due to damage to the central part of the retina, the lining of the eye, which produces a blurring of the central part of the visual field. The person with AMD often cannot recognize faces, though peripheral vision may survive.
- *Cataracts.* In much of the world, the clouding of the eye's crystalline lens is a leading cause of blindness. Initially, functional vision can be maintained using corrective lenses and good light, but as the cataracts further impair vision, surgery may be required.
- *Glaucoma.* Elevated pressure in the eye can lead to optic nerve damage, resulting in loss of peripheral vision, difficulty in focusing on objects, the presence of halos around lights, blurred vision, and eventually vision loss. Since the early stages are symptomless, many cases of progressive glaucoma go undiagnosed until it is too late to treat or restore vision.
- *Diabetic retinopathy.* A complication of diabetes, this condition occurs when blood vessels at the back of the eye are damaged. The cells of the retina die without proper nourishment, resulting in blind spots, blurring, and eventual blindness. People with either type-1 and type-2 diabetes are at risk of diabetic retinopathy.
- *Accidents.* Sports accidents, household chemicals, workshop and garden debris, battery acid, fireworks, overexposure to ultraviolet radiation, and other traumas to the eye produce visual impairments in countless people every year.

PREVENTION AND TREATMENT. A number of strategies can be employed to prevent or slow further vision loss.

- *Reduce eye strain.* Although general eye strain may not be a direct cause of vision loss, poor light, dry eyes, and prolonged computer use or television viewing can lead to headaches and stress and make your eyes more vulnerable to infections and irritation.

- *Use good lighting.* Proper kinds and amounts of light are essential to good vision. Needs vary, depending on the task being performed. During the aging years, we need approximately 10 percent more light with each passing decade.

- *Do exercises for your eyes.* Recent studies have found that aerobic exercise three times a week can reduce eye pressure (a major risk factor associated with glaucoma).

- *Consult your eye care professional regularly.* After age forty, see your ophthalmologist or optometrist every other year; after age sixty-five, annual visits are appropriate.

- *Respect warning signs.* Seek immediate care if you experience double or blurred vision or halos around lights; if you have difficulty distinguishing faces or print appears faded or distorted; if colors seem faded or washed out or floaters appear in your line of vision; if you bump into objects or have difficulty judging depth perception in climbing stairs; if your eyes adjust very slowing when going to light to dark; if you have sudden pain in one or both eyes.

- *Take care of your vision now.* Consume a varied diet with adequate vitamin C, vitamin E, beta-carotene, and zinc, nutrients essential to eye health. Wear eye protection when working with chemicals, power tools, and factory or construction equipment. Beware of the side effects of medications. Many prescription drugs, including some cold and allergy treatments, corticosteroids, certain heart medications, antidepressants, anticancer drugs, and others, may have side effects, especially for those at risk for glaucoma and cataracts. Consult your physician if you experience any problems.

- *Protect your eyes from ultraviolet rays.* UV light is short wavelength light beyond the visible spectrum. Exposure to UV sunlight, light reflected off water or snow, and strong artificial light such as tanning lamps can burn the surface of your eye in much the same way sunburn can damage the skin. Never look directly at the sun and wear UV-protective sunglasses that block 99 to 100 percent of UV rays.

Those shots we had as children? Some of the immunities established in our bodies back then are still working, but some are not. Other, newer immunizations have come into general use since then, some of which (like the flu shot) need to be given annually. In the interests of good health and longevity, you should be sure that your immunizations are up to date. Despite the debate about certain immunizations, the consensus is clear: The benefits outweigh the risks.

Shingles: *For whom and how often? A single vaccination, after age sixty.*
Formally known as *herpes zoster,* shingles is a painful skin eruption that tends to occur in older people (shingles strikes roughly a third of all adults). Caused by a reactivation of the same virus that causes chicken pox in children, shingles can also produce chronic and debilitating pain and, in some instances, eye involvement that results in vision loss.

Influenza: *For whom and how often? Most adults; annually, in the autumn*
The flu can be a deadly disease, particularly in older people; it is a viral infection that transforms from one year to the next, reaching peak prevalence in the winter months. In some years, the strain is more dangerous than others, but typically symptoms are chills, fever, sore throat, body aches, headache, cough, and general malaise. Pneumonia can follow.

Tetanus, Diphtheria, Pertussis (DTP) *For whom and how often? Tdap to age 64; TD among older adults; boosters thereafter of TD at ten-year intervals.*
Diphtheria (a throat infection that can lead to breathing problems and other complications), *pertussis* (whooping cough), and *tetanus* (lockjaw) are each caused by bacteria. The DTP vaccine was formulated to protect adolescents and adults from these diseases. Use is especially recommended when you expect to have close contact with children younger than twelve months of age.

Measles, Mumps, Rubella (MMR) *For whom and how often? One dose for adults born after 1957 is recommended.*
Although most people born prior to 1957 are generally considered to be immune to measles and mumps, younger adults should seek an MMR vaccination.

Pneumonia (PPV) *For whom and how often? At age sixty-five unless a previous inoculation was administered within last five years.*

Pneumococcal Polysaccharide vaccine protects against many varieties of the *Streptococcus pneumoniae* virus that can cause infections in the lungs (pneumonia), blood (bacteremia), and the covering of the brain (meningitis). People with special health problems such as alcoholism, heart or lung disease, kidney failure, diabetes, HIV infection, or certain cancers should be sure to keep their pneumonia inoculations up to date. The resistance of certain *pneumococcal* bacteria to penicillin and other drugs makes this even more important.

Other Vaccines *Hepatitis A* is recommended for certain individuals (including sexually active gay men and individuals who have sexual contact with intravenous drug users); *Varicella* (chicken pox) inoculations are appropriate for older people born outside of the United States.

Note: If your immune system is compromised, influenza and certain other so-called live vaccines are generally to be avoided. Discuss your circumstances with your physician.

For the most current information, check out the Centers for Disease Control recommendations at www.cdc.gov/vaccines/recs/schedules/adult-schedule.htm.

Anti-aging Drugs

With apologies to the editor of the New York *Sun* . . . No, Virginia, there is no anti-aging drug. Well, at least not yet, anyway.

That said, research is proceeding on many fronts to try to find the pharmacological fountain of youth, and agents that can slow, or even reverse, age-related degeneration seem increasingly possible. Among the other substances being investigated are:

Melatonin: The hormone melatonin is produced by the pineal gland in response to darkness. It plays a role in the body's daily (circadian) rhythms, as the levels of the melatonin rise prior to sleep. Synthetic melatonin has been used to treat sleep disorders, and substantial evidence exists of its utility in minimizing the effects of jet lag. There is also preliminary evidence that it may lower stress and enhance the immune system.

Despite some sensational claims made to the contrary, however, there is no evidence in humans that melatonin has any efficacy as an anti-aging remedy. Though available over the counter as a nonprescription dietary supplement in the United States, such sales are prohibited in Canada, Great Britain, and other European countries.

Human growth hormones: Produced by the pituitary gland (and, thanks to recombinant DNA technology, in the laboratory), HGH is widely promoted as an anti-aging agent. There is evidence that its use produces gains in muscle mass and skeletal density, as well as a decrease in fatty (adipose) tissue. There is no evidence that HGH enhances longevity (there is evidence, in fact, to the contrary in animal studies).

HGH is expensive and, to date, the only thing that is certain is that its marketers profit from its sale. It has important uses (especially in children whose bodies produce too little HGH), but its potential side effects suggest it is far from the anti-aging panacea that some of its purveyors claim. Buyer beware.

Testosterone. The male testes produce this hormone; production peaks in adolescence (it plays a vital role in puberty), while levels fall in the aging years. The decline is so gradual that there is substantial debate concerning so-called male menopause and what role testosterone does or does not play. In fact, the bodies of most men produce quantities of testosterone throughout life.

In men whose bodies produce no testosterone because of damaged testes or pituitary glands, testosterone replacement therapy strengthens muscles and bones and enhances sexual function. This, in part, has led to the various claims for testosterone therapy. However, the evidence for its potency in elderly men is unproven and many researchers believe, as well, that taking testosterone supplements may put men at greater risk for prostate cancer and perhaps even stroke because it stimulates the production of red blood cells.

While some older men who have tried testosterone supplementation report feeling younger, stronger, and having greater sexual potency, insufficient scientific research exists to demonstrate the benefits outweigh the potential risks.

Carnosine. This compound is found in the muscles and brain. Some bodybuilders take carnosine supplements in capsule form, believing it increases muscle strength and endurance. Other claims have been made for carnosine, among them that it has anticancer, anti-Alzheimer's, and antioxidant properties. As with many other dietary supplements, no clear scientific evidence exists that recommends its use as an agent of longevity.

Coenzyme Q10. Also known as CoQ10 and ubiquinone, this vitamin-like compound plays a role in the energy-producing function of healthy cells. There are early indications that it may be of use in treating the age-related eye disorder macular degeneration (see page 220), as an adjunct therapy in hypertension, and treating Alzheimer's disease, various heart problems, and numerous other disorders. While the future may hold much promise, the research findings remain preliminary. Discuss with your physician whether it might be of use to you (it has been increasingly prescribed for patients with heart failure).

Ginseng. The roots and leaves of this herb have, for thousands of years, been harvested, dried, and served as tea. Many claims have been made for the medicinal properties of the ginseng perennial plants *Panax ginseng* (Asian ginseng) and *P. quinquefolius* (American ginseng) as aphrodisiacs and stimulants. Ginseng has been said to improve memory, reduce feelings of stress, dissolve tumors, reverse aging, and deliver a wide range of other benefits.

If ginseng sounds too good be true, you are probably right. It is unlikely to prove to be the cure-all that some claim, although promising scientific findings suggest that ginseng may in fact boost the immune system, help control blood sugar levels, and be of use to heart patients. To be sure, additional studies are required.

For most people, though, ginseng poses little risk and promises modest potential health benefits (note, however, that the herb can have unwanted interactions in people taking oral diabetic medications and the blood thinner warfarin). There are dozens of ginseng preparations on the market in a wide range of doses, but as with all unproven medications, smaller quantities are to be preferred to megadoses.

Futureworld. Investigators are hopeful that activating the DNA enzyme telomerase might lead to life extension, but that remains in the realm of speculation. Stem cell research holds promise, too, but, again, much research remains to be done.

The Aging Driver

Older drivers have lots of experience, and virtues such as caution, good sense, and anticipation come with decades behind the wheel. But statistics also reveal that people over seventy-five are 37 percent more likely to have automobile accidents.

The years that brought us wisdom have also taken away some of our vision, hearing, and reaction time. In addition, older people are more likely to be taking medications that can cause drowsiness, to suffer from sleeplessness, and, in some cases, to experience disorientation and dementia.

All of which means there may come a time in our lives when it is the right thing to relinquish the keys to the car. For some people, it's a terrible prospect to contemplate: Many of us associate our independence, our ability to shop and socialize, and much else in our active lives, with getting behind the wheel. As a result, to be deprived of the ability to drive would require significant lifestyle adjustments.

Chronological age alone is no predictor of how well one drives. But there are certain physical and mental abilities that are required to drive well. If your skills have fallen below certain levels, you may have become a liability to yourself, your passengers, and anyone else on the road.

Loss of vision. Many states now mandate visions tests before renewing a driver's license. One can hardly argue with the reasoning: If you can't see what's in your path, you shouldn't be behind the wheel. If you require glasses to see distances, be sure to wear them when you drive. Does your vision no longer meet the minimum standard? That is, can you read a license plate, in good light, at a distance of five car lengths? If not, you need corrective lenses. Or to stop driving. Talk with your doctor or ophthalmologist.

Reduced night vision. The ability to see in reduced light diminishes with age; if your night vision is compromised, plan your life so you don't have to drive at night.

Physical impairments. If you have physical impairments—arthritis in your hands, for example, that makes managing the steering wheel difficult—there may be expedients. If your hearing is impaired, drive without the radio on and keep a window cracked in order to hear police and emergency vehicles. An automatic transmission, power steering, and power brakes can make things easier. If you have physical disabilities, an occupational therapist may be able to suggest solutions. But if you don't feel you can safely handle the two-ton machine that is your car, don't drive.

Be honest with yourself. Have you recently had an accident in which you were found at fault? Are you regularly surprised at the sudden appearance of a pedestrian or another car in your path? Do you sometimes feel confused at intersections? Are you easily distracted from the complex tasks of driving? Are you inconsistent in controlling your speed (perhaps you start out going very slowly, but sometimes find yourself racing along much than faster than you intended)? Do people seem to be honking at you more often than they used to do? Do you have trouble maneuvering your head and shoulders to see around you? Do you drive over curbs sometimes? Do you regularly get lost in familiar neighborhoods?

Any of these may signal that it's time to turn in the keys. In fact, there is pending legislation in several states to require both vision and road tests before renewing the licenses of people of advanced age, so the state may make the decision for you.

On the other hand, there may be expedients you can employ to keep you on the road—and safe. Allow yourself space: On the highway don't tailgate, in a parking lot find the biggest space to pull into. Slow down a little: By reducing your speed, you increase your time to react to situations. Do one thing at a time (that is, drive), and don't distract yourself from the task by talking, eating, drinking, or using your cell phone. Find your comfort zone: That may mean avoiding rush hour, staying off highways, keeping out of midtown, not driving in inclement weather, avoiding long-distance driving, or never driving alone.

If the time has come to turn in the keys, however, just do it. If you are concerned with the diminished abilities of another member of your family and you find it difficult to confront the older person, talk to his or her physician. That is a role the doctor should be willing to take.

Life can be lived fully even without a car. You might be surprised at how many solutions there are to getting where you want to go.

Strategy Twenty-three: Investigate the Internet

The Internet seems to offer just about everything: products, services, and information on a bewildering array of subjects in essentially all the languages of the world. You can make friends, conduct business, search for a lost high school classmate, read a book, apply to college, get the most current stock prices—and find health and medical advice.

THE ASSIGNMENT. Acquaint—or better acquaint—yourself with the wealth of possibilities for information on the Internet.

1. To gain knowledge and perspective, learn how to search and find information sources on the Web.
2. Incorporate the Internet into your life to stimulate your brain, to enhance your social network.
3. Be a little skeptical as you collect information on the Web. There are charlatans and profiteers, as well as countless legitimate sources of knowledge and products. (See also *Navigating the News*, page 10.)

THE POSSIBILITIES. Truly there is something for everyone out there, whether you are buying or selling, learning or teaching, whether your taste runs to the old-fashioned or the newfangled. And the Web really is easy to access once you have a little basic knowledge.

- *Find a mentor.* If you have no computer experience, you would be wise to find a mentor to get you started. It may be a friend or family member (grandkids are often the best; to them, working on a computer is second nature). If you have the means, you may find that paying a professional by the hour is your best bet, since you're hiring them to be patient with you as you take some baby steps. Whoever is to be your guide, remember that there is no such thing as a stupid question.
- *Get access to a computer.* You will need a computer. You may not have to buy one; to start with, you may find using someone else's makes the process less daunting. Or use one at the local public library. If you decide to acquire your own, the choices are a laptop (it's about the size of a loose-leaf binder) or a desktop (it consists of separate components, including a TV screen monitor, keyboard,

and a metal box of the electronic bits and pieces, which is called the CPU, or central processing unit). Formerly laptops commanded premium prices, but that isn't so true any longer, and they're portable. But look at the choices and decide what suits your needs.

- *Connect to the Internet.* Your means of access to the Internet may be via a modem connected to your phone lines (spend the extra dollars per months for broadband; the old basic phone line connection probably will be so slow as to be very frustrating) or wireless (meaning you'll need another piece of hardware called a router that broadcasts the signal to its immediate environment). Your cable provider may be another option for service. Again, your mentor can guide you through what seems a complicated setup process but is really very routine.

- *Start with what you know.* Once you're equipped and ready to venture out onto the World Wide Web, explore territory about which you know something. Using one of the search engines (Google .com is the dominant name in the market at the moment), type in a keyword in the empty box. It might be *chess* or *Lapsang Souchong* or *Harry Potter.* You will be offered a range of Internet destinations. Try out a few them; just click your mouse on top of one, and you're off on a journey.

- *Expand your universe.* You can literally look at the universe through the Hubble telescope, visit national parks, or learn more than you ever wanted to know about the movies of Humphrey Bogart. The next time you have a question you can't answer about raising chickens—or anything else—the answer is probably somewhere on the Web. You can sign up (mostly for free) to get full-text access to the world's best newspapers, and even get breaking news sent to you by e-mail. Looking to buy a new book or a belt or an alarm clock? Almost every retailer today has a website. If you're looking to buy something old or used, there's always ebay.com and other similar sites. If you're looking for a job, services, or all kinds of goods, there's craigslist.com. There are even places that offer tutorials on using the net, such as learnthenet.com.

- *Join a social network.* There are a great many compatible people out there, walking the gossamer of silicon threads that is the World Wide Web. That means that they are people to talk to. The terms of contact are different, but in a matter of minutes you will find that chatting online isn't so strange. And all of a sudden a new route to exchanging ideas, trading stories, and getting to know new people opens to you. (For more on social networking, see *The Society of Cyberspace*, page 128.)

- *Be a little bit wary of what you learn.* When it comes to gathering information, judge the source. Typically you will find some authoritative and respected institutions alongside unfamiliar organizations that make claims that you suspect (or perhaps know) to be exaggerated. How can you distinguish one from the other? Here are few guidelines. Have you ever heard of the organization? Is it a dot.com or a dot.edu? (The former is likely to be profit-seeking, the latter a university.) Are the claims or data presented original to the source or a report of someone else's research? As with other media, go to the primary source if possible. Check the date, since the Internet can be a time warp: Old pages (called "zombies") that remain unrevised may be offering information that is badly outdated. If the claims made lead to a sales pitch or if the website is associated with a new product, advertiser, or corporation, the information may have a commercial bias. When it comes to anything that might prompt you to action—a buying decision, a medical judgment, a financial option—keep in mind that the virtual world of the Web is like real life. Do not take one claim as the final truth. Look to learn more from other sites and sources; in effect, get a second opinion.

- *Be an explorer.* You needn't just settle for e-mail or an occasional check-in at a few favorite sites. You can venture far afield, seeking not only friends but travel opportunities, all sorts of knowledge, and ideas about planning your future. The Internet can be informative, rewarding . . . and just plain fun.

Strategy Twenty-four: Be a Good Patient

Would you be glad to see yourself coming through the door? If you are the sort of patient you would dread seeing, you need to change some things.

THE ASSIGNMENT. Navigating the doctor's office.

1. Imagine yourself in the doctor's or the nurse's shoes.
2. Speak in a way that you would want to be spoken to: with respect, consideration, and an eye on getting what you want because the medical professionals want to please you.

THE TECHNIQUES. Try one or more of these approaches.

- *Act like a salesman.* People in sales learn the rule early: You want the attention of a decider? Be nice to his or her assistant. The odds of your call getting through, of getting access, vary directly with how much the gatekeeper wants to help you. The same is true with nurses.
- *If possible, smile.* There is scientific evidence that smiles beget smiles in this life, and that is probably even more the case in charged interactions like those between caregivers and patients.
- *Balance niceness and necessity.* There is fine line between acceptance and activism. The best patient is the one who comes with intelligent questions. The patient, whether in excellent health or suffer-

ing with an ailment, should not merely accept everything the doctor says as the incontrovertible truth. You need to understand why a particular treatment is warranted; if you are presented with a choice, your decision should be made on the basis of all the facts.

- *Watch out for yourself, too.* People often seek careers in health care because they have a desire to serve others. That said, in an environment where the demands are unending, the staff insufficient, and the hours long—unfortunately that describes the average hospital—not every doctor, nurse, orderly, or other member of the staff can focus their best attention on every patient. That means you need to be very much on top of your care.

- *Use your deputies.* Your spouse, partners, children, or others in your inner circles have roles to play, too, as details get forgotten or overlooked in even the best doctor's offices and hospitals.

- *Find a doctor you trust.* He or she will be your partner in safeguarding your health.

- *Educate yourself.* When it comes to the preventive strategies your doctor proposes—the work you need to do to lose weight, exercise more, quit smoking or drinking, to reduce stress—find the time and self-discipline to do it.

- *Obey orders.* Your physician can play a role in enhancing your longevity, but only if you let him or her. A good working partnership with your doctor and other health care providers can help you change your bad habits, but you need to take the advice you are given seriously. If your doctor prescribes medication to control your blood pressure or lower your cholesterol, you need to use it as prescribed. If your physician advises that you lose a few pounds, recommends you start exercising, orders you to limit your consumption of alcohol, insists you stop smoking, or asks you to make other lifestyle changes, find a way to do as you are told. Unlike one of your grade school teachers, your doctor cannot punish you with a poor grade for homework refusal. But in failing to follow doctor's orders, you will be punishing yourself.

Diabetes in the Aging Years

Diabetes—more precisely diabetes mellitus—is a disorder in which the body fails to properly metabolize blood sugar (glucose). The mechanism for managing this essential source of energy for your cells is the hormone insulin, which is produced by the pancreas. In people with diabetes, either the supply of insulin is insufficient or the cells have become resistant to insulin. The result is, in effect, the same: too much glucose in the body. Too much blood sugar can pose an immediate health risk; in the long term, complications can develop involving the kidneys, eyes, blood vessels, and nervous system.

Type-1 diabetes, sometimes referred to the now outmoded terms *insulin-dependent diabetes* and *juvenile diabetes*, usually occurs before age thirty. It is the result of an autoimmune reaction in which the body damages the insulin-producing cells in the pancreas. With the pancreas no longer able to produce insulin, regular injections are required for the body to process blood sugars normally.

Roughly nine in ten diabetics have type-2 diabetes, and most of them are diagnosed after age forty. Although the pancreas continues to produce insulin, the hormone has difficulty accessing passageways into the cells of the person with type-2 diabetes. Thus the glucose remains in the bloodstream, and the pancreas reacts by releasing more insulin.

SYMPTOMS. The classic signs of diabetes are an insatiable thirst and increased urination. Blurred vision, recurrent vaginal yeast infections, skin infections, and an overall sense of malaise may also be indicators. Weight loss can occur, despite increased appetite and food consumption. In many people with type-2 diabetes, however, the symptoms may be so subtle that years pass before they are recognized.

Exercise and diet. If your physician identifies elevated glucose levels in your blood, the first avenue of approach is likely to be regular aerobic exercise. Exercise stimulates the pancreas and may well help you avoid the need to take oral diabetic medications. A balanced diet is important, too, and you will be given detailed instructions about the consumption of complex carbohydrates (starches) and the exclusion of the simple sugars of sweets.

Prevention. There are no guarantees, but if you or your doctor are concerned that you might develop diabetes (see *Are You at Risk of Diabetes?*, below), the single best strategy for prevention is regular exercise. Exercise burns calories and helps control weight. It enhances insulin action and lowers blood glucose. The possibility of developing diabetes is yet another reason to establish a regular exercise program (see *Prescription VI: Live the Active Life*, page 138). For the person already diagnosed with diabetes, the usual prescription is a regime of regular exercise, strict adherence to a diabetic diet, attention to glucose monitoring, and appropriate use of oral diabetic medications.

are you at risk of diabetes?

In the aging years, some people are at greater risk for diabetes than others. These factors may predispose you to diabetes:

- Obesity (see *Body Mass Index*, page 141)
- Hypertension in excess of 140/90 mm Hg (see *Managing Your Blood Pressure*, page 246)
- A sedentary lifestyle that involves little physical activity
- A family history of diabetes, especially a parent or sibling
- A history of gestational diabetes during pregnancy or delivery of a baby that weighed more than nine pounds
- Membership in a high-risk group for diabetes (such as Native American, African-American, or Latino)

- Low HDL cholesterol levels or high triglycerides
- Impaired glucose tolerance

If you are at risk, focus on the factors you can change (your weight and inactivity) and those you can manage (blood pressure and blood lipid levels). By taking a proactive approach you may be able to exercise control over your blood sugar, avoid the need for diabetic medications, and avoid the potential health impacts of diabetes. Your good efforts to work out more often, eat better, and manage your existing health problems can enhance your longevity.

Cancer Prevention

Cancer used to be one of the most feared words in the language, but the sharp edge of terror that the word once produced has been dulled because so many cancers have become survivable diseases. We all know people who, their cancers cured, have resumed ordinary lives with normal life expectancies. Some types of cancers have become lifestyle diseases that one lives with for many years, just as people do with diabetes, arthritis, and high blood pressure. A cancer diagnosis today means choices, strategies, and, very often, a return to good health.

Our focus here, however, is on *avoiding* cancer, on doing everything you can to help ensure you do not hear the word "cancer" applied to you. An emerging body of knowledge suggests that decisions we make about how we live our lives can affect our risk of developing many cancers. The older we are, the greater is our cumulative exposure to carcinogens such as air pollutants, radiation, and the sun's rays, but there are steps we can take to avoid or minimize our exposure. Years of bad habits can predispose us to certain cancers, but we can decide to consume less alcohol, stop smoking, and eat low-fat diets, all of which will reduce our risk for cancer. Stress reduction, too, may make us less likely to hear our physician utter the once dreaded diagnosis.

Cancer is actually a group of related diseases. Normal cells in the body grow and divide in an orderly way to serve the body's needs, but when certain cells in the body begin to divide and multiply in an uncontrolled way, the result can be an unwanted mass of tissue called a *tumor*.

Tumors are divided into two basic categories, *malignant* and *benign*. Benign tumors are not cancerous; they can be removed and, in most cases, neither recur nor spread to other parts of the body. Malignant tumors, however, are cancers that invade nearby tissues. When a malignancy spreads (*metastasizes*) through the bloodstream or lymphatic system, it can damage tissues remote from the original site. Most cancers are named for their point of origin (lung cancer, skin cancer, liver cancer, and so on), but there are also cancers called leukemia and lymphoma that occur in blood-forming cells.

PREVENTION. The complexities of cancer are many. Heredity is one factor. In some families, for example, cancer of the breast occurs much more frequently than in the general population. There are evident links between the occurrence of certain cancers and the way we live our lives. Here lung cancer is the most obvious example: Some 85 percent of those who die of lung cancer were smokers. The more you smoke, the longer you smoke, and the deeper you inhale, the more likely you are to face a lung cancer diagnosis.

Some risk factors for cancer cannot be avoided (you cannot choose your parents), others can be (you can elect to quit smoking). As new understandings of the mechanism, causes, and course of cancers emerge, there are more preventive strategies you may wish to contemplate.

Tobacco. This is an obvious case, since smoking cigarettes, pipes, or cigars puts you at increased risk for not only lung cancer but cancers of the mouth, throat, larynx, esophagus, stomach, liver, prostate, colon, rectum, pancreas, bladder, kidney, and cervix. Smokeless tobacco increases your risk of cancers of the mouth and throat.

If you are a smoker, stop. Now. Even if you have smoked for many years, the chances of contracting lung cancer drop when you stop; statistics suggest that after fifteen years, former smokers have a risk of lung cancer that approaches that of people who have never smoked. On the other hand, the odds of a one-pack-a-day smoker contracting lung cancer is *ten times* greater than that of nonsmokers.

Alcohol. Heavy drinkers put themselves at increased risk of liver, oral, esophageal, and breast cancer; that risk is substantially higher still for drinkers who also smoke. Drink in moderation or not at all (see *Alcohol: Tonic or Toxin?*, page 193).

Diet and weight control. Obesity and certain dietary habits have also been associated with higher risks of breast, colorectal, uterine, pancreatic, ovarian, and prostate cancers. As a result, the National Cancer Institute recommends a low-fat diet, one with only modest amounts of red meat, eggs, oils, and high-fat dairy products (whole milk, butter, and cheese). On other hand, you should consume quantities of whole-grain foods, fruits, and vegetables. That will mean you are ingesting generous amounts of vitamins, minerals, and fiber, which are believed to offer some protective effects.

Sun exposure. Sustained exposure to the sun, particularly when the sun is high in the sky, is to be avoided. Sunscreen is a second essential strategy: Apply it to any and all exposed skin well before sun exposure (a good plan is to make it a daily step in your morning ablutions). The measure of how much protection a given product offers is indicated by its *SPF* (sun protective factor), which should be noted on the packaging. A minimum of 15 SPF is recommended, although pale-complexioned people, particularly those with red hair or who tend to freckle, should use a sunscreen with a SPF of 25 or more.

Other strategies. Good overall physical conditioning is a factor in enhancing longevity: regular exercise, stress management, adequate sleep, and an engaged life can also help you be and stay healthy.

cancer symptoms

Cancer often has no symptoms; on the other hand, there are certain signs that, if you detect them, should be cause for investigation. Consult your physician if you experience:

- A thickening of tissue or a lump in your breast or anywhere else
- Unexplained weight loss

- Skin sores that do not heal, a mole or wart that undergoes changes
- Unusual bleeding or discharge
- Difficulty swallowing or white patches in the mouth
- A nagging cough or hoarseness
- Unfamiliar and unexplained pain
- Changes in bowel habits or function
- Extreme fatigue or lingering fever

If you observe any of these symptoms, do not assume you have cancer, since any and all may well be caused by many other conditions, most of them minor. However, see your doctor to get the symptoms evaluated.

Laughter Is the Best Medicine

Laughter is a happy surprise. According to cardiologists at the University of Maryland Medical Center in Baltimore, it may also have some protective effects in the battle against heart disease.

The Maryland researchers selected three hundred people. Half had had a cardiac event or bypass surgery; the others were healthy with no indications of heart disease. All the volunteers completed two questionnaires, one of which sought to determine how much (or how little) the volunteers laughed in response to certain stimuli. The other looked to measure hostility or anger. The findings were intriguing: The volunteers with heart disease were 40 *percent* less likely to laugh in a variety of situations compared to people of the same age without heart disease.

Lead researcher Michael Miller, M.D., summarized the finding this way: "The ability to laugh—either naturally or as learned behavior—may have important implications in societies such as the U.S. where heart disease remains the number one killer."

Several years later, he conducted a follow-up study in which healthy participants watched portions of two movies, one violent and stressful, the other funny and light. Reporting his findings in 2005, Miller found that in almost three-fourths of the subjects, the protective inner lining of their blood vessels, the endothelium, constricted during the viewing of the intense movie. In contrast, in more than 90 percent of the volunteers the blood vessels relaxed during the laughter-inducing film. In numerical terms, the study found that average blood flow increased 22 percent during laughter and decreased 35 percent during mental stress.

End-of-Life Decisions

Many doctors remain hesitant to broach the subject of death, but in an effort to exercise some control over your life in the face of a potentially terminal disease, the subject can hardly be ignored. You need some best-guess estimates of your prognosis as you move forward. You may also be surprised to learn how matter of fact the conversation can be once it has begun. Among the questions you may wish to ask are these:

- *What are the chances I can be cured?*
- *Will surgery, chemotherapy, or other proposed treatments extend my life?*
- *Are there experimental therapies or trials that might offer new promise?*
- *What will my quality of life be as a consequence of the treatments?*
- *What will be the side effects of treatment?*
- *What is my likely life expectancy?*
- *What are the costs and how much will my insurance cover?*

If the prospects of a cure appear high, if quality of life can be maintained, or the treatments offer promise for extending your life, the decision to proceed with a recommended treatment regimen may be easy.

On the other hand, if the news isn't so optimistic, the answers to these questions may be hard to hear. The will to live is in the nature of our species, but not everyone responds to a given set of facts in the same way. Some people choose to fight even in the face of seemingly insurmountable odds; others simply resign themselves to their fate. There may be a middle ground, too, involving palliative chemotherapy that can offer some short-term benefit and a time to find closure.

The decision to proceed with intensive therapies is yours to make, but keep in mind that there is something physicians call futile care; they are treatments that are more likely to harm than to help a patient. So if your physician can offer no rosy promises, you may choose not to proceed with all-out attempts at a cure but opt instead for palliative care in which the goals become pain control and your comfort. The acceptance of such an approach raises a set of nonmedical questions you may need to address, such as:

- *Do I need to execute or update my will?*
- *Should I be setting up a trust or other legal arrangement to facilitate the resolution of my affairs?*
- *Do I wish to have a do-not-resuscitate (DNR) order in place?*
- *With whom do I need to share news of my illness?*
- *Are there other financial or legal issues (such as durable power of attorney) that need to be resolved?*

A third and equally crucial battery of questions may come next. These concern your peace of mind and coping with the fear and other emotional burdens of facing a terminal illness. Some of these are questions for you to ponder alone, while others may lead to important discussions with loved ones.

- *Should I open a dialogue with a spiritual or psychological advisor?*
- *In making decisions, do I need to set up a decision tree to establish priorities for my spouse, partner, children, physicians, and caregivers?*
- *What arrangements need to be made for my care and respite care for loved ones who will be helping during my illness?*
- *How will I spend my remaining time?*
- *How do I tell my family and friends?*
- *What has my life meant to me and to others? (See* Life Review, *page 43.)*

No one wants to contract a terrible disease or hear that his or her life will soon end, but many dying people find they inhabit a new and peaceful plane after acceptance of the harsh facts; their remaining days can become a time of forgiveness, a time to express feelings, thanks, regret, and even joy.

Among survivors there is often a surprising sense that the disease has made them stronger or better human beings. Dr. Jerri Nielsen's perspective on cancer is important in this context. She was the physician who, while stationed at the South Pole, diagnosed her own breast cancer. She felt she was better for the experience of cancer: "We're not on Earth to see how long we can live," Nielsen said after her ordeal. "We should look for peace in chaos and contentment in disaster. It's also important to learn that people need each other. I didn't save myself [in Antarctica]; I was saved by others."

the health care proxy

When we are healthy, it may be difficult to imagine the need to delegate to another person the responsibility for making life-and-death decisions. Yet, in order to be sure your wishes are respected in the event of a health care crisis, it is important to execute a legal document that designates to whom the doctors will turn in the event you are not capable of making your own decisions.

Health Care Proxy

1. I, _____ residing at

_____

(Street) (City or Town) (State)

hereby appoint as my Health Care Agent:

_____

(Name of person you choose as Agent)

of _____.

(Street) (City/Town) (State) (Phone)

If my Agent is unwilling or unable to serve, then I appoint as my Alternate Agent:

_____

(Name of person you choose as Alternate Agent)

of _____ .

(Street) (City/Town) (State) (Phone)

2. My Agent shall have the authority to make all health care decisions for me, including decisions about life-sustaining treatment, subject to any limitations I
state below, if I am unable to make health care decisions myself. My Agent's
authority becomes effective if my attending physician determines in writing
that I lack the capacity to make or to communicate health care decisions. My
Agent is then to have the same authority to make health care decisions as I
would if I had the capacity to make them

EXCEPT _____

_____ .

(List of limitations)

I direct my Agent to make health care decisions based on my Agent's assessment of my personal wishes. If my personal wishes are unknown, my Agent is
to make health care decisions based on my Agent's assessment of my best
interests. Photocopies of this Health Care Proxy shall have the same force
and effect as the original and may be given to other health care providers.

3. **Signed:**

[Complete only if Principal is physically unable to sign]:
I have signed the Principal's name above at his/her direction in the presence
of the Principal and two witnesses.

_____

(Name)

_____ .

(Street) (City/Town) (State)

4. **WITNESS STATEMENT:** We, the undersigned, each witnessed the sign-
ing of this Health Care Proxy by the Principal or at the direction of the Principal and state that the Principal appears to be at least 18 years of age, of
sound mind and under no constraint or undue influence. Neither of us is
named as the Health Care Agent or Alternate Agent in this document.

In our presence, on this day of _____ , 20 _____ .

Witness #1: _____ .
                              (Signature)

Name *(print)*: _____ .

_____ .
                    (Street) (City/Town) (State)

Witness #2: _____ .
                              (Signature)

Name *(print)*: _____ .

_____ .
                    (Street) (City/Town) (State)

The above is a basic boilerplate for your reference, but you should seek out a form that is legal in your state.

Heart and Vascular Disease

The heart is a muscular organ that pumps blood to your cells. It does so via the vascular system, the network of blood vessels that decreases in size from the aorta to the arteries, arterioles, and capillaries. Together, the heart and the vascular system constitute a remarkable circulatory mechanism that functions as few man-made machines can. Essentially every second of your life, a contraction of the heart muscle sends the life-giving oxygen and nutrients to the farthest reaches of your body. When the action of the heart stops, life ceases in a matter of minutes.

During the aging years in particular, the cardiovascular system may begin to function less efficiently. Heart output decreases after age thirty, and blood vessels begin to stiffen and narrow, meaning the heart has to work harder. The aging heart develops thicker walls from having to do the extra work. This results in higher blood pressure. When the blood pressure rises to unhealthy levels, it is called *hypertension*; one in three Americans has high blood pressure, which is a leading cause of stroke, heart failure, and heart attack. A significant narrowing of the arteries around the heart is called *coronary artery disease*; the cause is usually *atherosclerosis*, in which fatty deposits called plaque, which consist of cholesterol-rich plaque and calcium, accumulate on the blood vessel linings. This increases the risk of blockage of a coronary artery (*myocardial ischemia*), which can, in turn, produce chest pain (*angina*) or even the death of heart tissue (*myocardial infarction*). The cumulative effects of hypertension, atherosclerosis, heart attack, or other conditions may impair the pumping capacity of the heart, resulting in *congestive heart failure*. When an artery in the brain becomes blocked or ruptures, the result is *stroke*, a medical emergency that interrupts brain function because the flow of blood to the cells of the brain is interrupted. Not all strokes are the same: some are *ischemic*, meaning an artery is blocked, usually by a blood clot; others are *hemorrhagic*, in which a blood vessel bursts, flooding surrounding brain tissue with blood.

All of this adds up to the fact that, taken together, heart and blood vessel diseases are the number one killer by far in the United States every year.

Yet that daunting fact should be seen in counterpoint to happier news about health trends, research, and prevention of cardiovascular disease. The rate of death from heart disease among men and women between twenty-five and eighty-four dropped by about 50 percent between 1980 and 2000. About half of the improvement is attributable to improved treatments for people with existing heart problems, but much of the rest is thought to be the result of a reduction of key risk factors for heart disease. These include lower cholesterol levels, better blood pressure management, decreased smoking, and increases in physical activity.

PREVENTING HEART DISEASE. When it comes to heart disease and vascular disease in most of its guises, a healthy lifestyle is, once again, a big factor in your longevity.

Quit smoking. I have said it before and will again: To smoke is to endanger your health, and when it comes to coronary artery disease, the toll taken by smoking is great.

Control your hypertension. The discovery that you have hypertension should be interpreted as a call to action. If the diagnosis of this medical condition is not good news, it does offer the opportunity to change your habits and slow or even reverse the harm that high blood pressure can do to your blood vessels, heart, and other organs. See *Managing Your Blood Pressure*, below.

Reduce your blood lipids. America's obsession with cholesterol is undeniable; while perhaps oversimplified, a high cholesterol level, particularly of LDL (low-density lipoprotein), is a risk factor for heart disease, as are elevated levels of another blood fat called triglycerides. Levels of total cholesterol over 200 milligrams per deciliter are regarded as elevated; those above 240 high. LDL over 130 is borderline high, above 160 high; with triglycerides, elevated is above 150, high is over 200.

If you have excess blood fats, you and your physician should discuss the appropriate approach. A reduction of fats in the diet is usually an essential part of a cholesterol-lowering strategy (see *Prescription VII: Eat Your Way to Health*, page 179); exercise, too, can help lower cholesterol (see *Prescription VI: Live the Active Life*, page 138). Depending upon your family history, your use of alcohol and tobacco, whether or not you are overweight (see *Strategy Thirteen: Determine Your Body Mass Index*, page 141), and your overall health status, the use of a cholesterol-lowering drug may be appropriate, too.

Get some exercise. Physical activity may be the single most important determinant in maintaining heart health. The heart is, after all, a muscle; exercising it to keep it in good condition is invaluable. Even if you have had a cardiac event, an appropriate program of exercise can help restore you to good health. However, before embarking on a vigorous exercise program, consult your physician, especially if you are overweight; if you have a significant health issue (such as diabetes or heart, lung, or kidney disease); or there is a family history of heart or vascular disease.

managing your blood pressure

Blood pressure is a dual measure of the pressure exerted by the flow of blood to the major vessels that delivers the blood to the body. Your blood pressure reading reflects the maximum pressure ("systolic," pronounced *sis-TALL-ik*) and minimum pressure ("diastolic," as in *dye-ess-TALL-ik*) that are exerted on artery walls during the heart's pumping cycle. It is rendered in conversational speech as, for example, "one-twenty over eighty" (120/80); that's shorthand for 120 millimeters of mercury (mmHg).

High blood pressure is a bit like carbon monoxide. Our senses are unable to detect either one: Hypertension has no symptoms, and CO, a normal by-product of combustion, has no taste, smell, or color. The stealthy nature of both makes them especially dangerous. When inhaled, CO starves the body of oxygen, potentially resulting in death; untreated hypertension can lead to serious health problems, including stroke, heart disease, kidney failure, and loss of eyesight. The absence of evident symptoms is one reason hypertension is often called the silent killer.

By age sixty-five, your risk of developing hypertension is 50 percent. Diet and stress appear to be causative factors (the role of aging is less certain), but maintaining normal blood pressure (that is, a reading of 120/80 or below) is important.

Not all hypertension is the same. One variety, *isolated systolic hypertension* (ISH) is characterized by elevated systolic pressure (greater than 160 mmHg) but with nearly normal diastolic pressure (typically in the range of 90 mmHg). This type of hypertension is typically treated with inexpensive diuretics, drugs that reduce the amount of water retained by body.

The second variety of high blood pressure is more dangerous because both systolic and diastolic pressures are elevated. The classifications of hypertension are thus determined by the pressures, and are as follows:

- *Normal:* A blood pressure reading of less than 120/80
- *Prehypertensive or High Normal:* Between 120 and 139 systolic, or between 80 and 89 diastolic
- *High Blood Pressure (Stage I):* Between 140 and 159 systolic, or 90 and 99 diastolic
- *High Blood Pressure (Stage II):* Over 159 systolic or 100 diastolic

Many people can control their hypertension by means of lifestyle changes; rather than taking pills on a daily basis, it is preferable to establish a new exercise routine, to eat sensibly, and identify strategies for lessening the stress in your life. In instances where your blood pressure is unacceptably high or changes in behavior prove insufficient, your physician has a wide range of pharmaceutical treatments from which to choose.

Even in the absence of apparent symptoms, elevated blood pressure is a danger to your health. Bringing the pressure down to normal limits is important—and achievable.

PRESCRIPTION VIII

YOUR THREE STRATEGIES TO PRACTICING PREVENTION

At the core of this chapter is a three-step prescription for you to take an active role in managing your own care.

Strategy Twenty-two: Master the Medical Tests
Your doctor relies upon them—and you should know what they mean, too. See page 212.

Strategy Twenty-three: Investigate the Internet
Knowledge is a useful tool; the World Wide Web puts a vast amount of information only a few clicks away. See page 228.

Strategy Twenty-four: Be a Good Patient
Do unto your medical caregivers as you would have done unto you. See page 232.

If you practice prevention, you increase your odds of living longer.

PRESCRIPTION IX

STAY WITH
THE STRATEGY

❖

RECOGNIZING THE NEED FOR HEALTHY CHANGE IS ESSENTIAL.
Your body may pose challenges you cannot afford to ignore. The onset of
diabetes or heart problems, for example, may make certain bad habits you
have long recognized no longer deniable. Your physician may tell you that
your very survival depends on making changes. But the recognition is of
value only if you do something about it.

On the other hand, you probably are aware of issues that you need to
address in advance of any such medical alarms. The person who continues
to smoke in the face of an avalanche of evidence about tobacco's detrimen-
tal health effects is feigning deafness to a very loud alarm. People who get
little or no exercise, those who make no attempt lose excess pounds, and
individuals who drink excessive quantities of alcohol are effectively adding
years to their chronological age by disposing themselves to disorders that af-

fect a disproportionate number of people who are overweight, inactive, or alcoholic. A growing body of evidence suggests that intellectual lethargy—the failure to exercise your cognitive abilities—is a factor in mental decline in the aging years.

Let's acknowledge a simple fact: All of us can make changes to enhance our health, to ensure that we can make the most of the three-decade dividend. The goal of this closing chapter is to help you shape (or reshape) strategies to make such changes. In earlier chapters, I've talked about the science, about the investigators who are looking at longevity. But now I am asking you to focus primarily on your own life. That was a question we asked of Rachel.

Rachel's Healthy Day

"Tell us about your average day," we instructed respondents in a recent questionnaire. Some people gave us a few words, others a few sentences, but one (we'll call her Rachel) was thorough in filling us in about her day.

Rachel is sixty-nine (going on forty-nine, it seems) and in good health. Although she was revered during her many years as a teacher and principal at an independent school, her life has not been especially remarkable: college, teaching, marriage, children, some community service, being a principal, retirement. She has a husband and two daughters and resides in suburban New York. A very good life, all in all, and one that, as you will see, has been enlivened by the zest (and good sense) she invests in it.

This is her response:

"*Mornings*. After a good night's sleep—I'm lucky, I know, to be a good sleeper—I awake refreshed. Every day is a small gift (my dad died at fifty-one; I've never really gotten over that), so I take a deep breath and try to think one thought of something that makes me happy. It might be a memory, a friend's face, or, I don't know, the fact that lots of young boys got enthusiastic about reading because of Harry Potter. It's a good way to start the day. Then I pat Bill on the rump—my husband's generally still asleep at six o'clock. He usually grunts, and we may exchange a few words as I do a few easy stretching exercises. A little bit of arthritis is creeping into my joints, and the stretches really help get me going.

"My morning ablutions are probably like most people's, but I'm religious about brushing and flossing my teeth and using sunscreen (my doctor recently gave me a big talking-to about that!). Breakfast? I'm a tea drinker, so I make a pot. I like hot whole-grain cereals, fruit, and juice. One of my daughters got me in the habit of using low-fat milk, but I still miss the half-and-half I used to use. I take a multivitamin and a couple of other supplements, including calcium. They can't hurt, right?

"Three days a week I go to the community center downtown and help prepare and package hot dinners for Meals On Wheels. I do not have much to do with the cooking—though they sometimes use an old family recipe I shared with them—but there is a lot of dishing up, bagging, and labeling to do. I'm a pretty organized person, so on the days I'm there, I usually try to do the last check of the boxes before the delivery people leave.

"*Afternoons*. I'm almost always done by lunch. Lately, Bill and I usually have been meeting at the new bagel place, but sometimes he plays golf. I never have trouble finding somebody to have lunch with, though; I've lived in this town a long time. I avoid the cream cheese, of course, though I used to like a schmear on my bagel, but they always have some kind of sandwich filling that is not too heavy on the mayo.

"The afternoon is my time. At least one afternoon a week I try to expose myself to something new. Our local art museum is my favorite stop, but sometimes it's a movie or I take the train into New York City for a show or to visit one of the museums there. Or just walk in the park. During the growing season, though, I spend time in my garden a few days a week. I know pulling up weeds and pruning and planting bulbs and wielding that shovel help keep me in some kind of shape. Most afternoons I treat myself to a short nap (twenty minutes will usually do it). And almost every day I spend some time reading a book. I do not think of that as a luxury; that's my reward for those years of work. I've recently finished rereading all of Jane Austen and now I'm moving on to Anthony Trollope (now there is a big assignment!). Oh, and then there's the walk. Often with Bill, half an hour or so, before I make dinner.

"*Evenings*. I like to cook, especially since I retired and have the time to do it right. With Bill's heart attack ten years ago, we've had to be really good about eating carefully. A trip we took to Italy introduced us to polenta and risotto. Most of our dinners have almost no red meat and often only a little chicken or fish. Bill's a little bit proud of his salad making and of his vegetable garden, so we are good that way, too. He likes a glass of red wine (well, two, but rarely more), and he usually reads the paper while I cook. Sometimes I'll have wine, too, but it has to be white. The red no longer agrees with me.

"Our lives are pretty quiet. Bill still bowls in a league, and I go to both the women's club and the historical society at least once a month in the evenings. He does the top half of the crossword puzzle and leaves me the bottom half every night. We have a couple of shows we like on TV; not every night but several nights a week. And the girls each call every few days, usually after dinner. I wish they were closer; California's too far away, but we do make at least two trips a year there and they come and visit every summer (both girls are teachers, I'm proud to say). Bill and I still enjoy each other's company in all the right ways, too, if you know what I mean.

"I'm sure this is not what you expected—too much, right? But I couldn't help myself."

No, Rachel, it is not too much at all. It has so many good ingredients for longevity, it has the distinct echo of good sense.

Setting the Stage for Change

Aging is not an overnight event. We do not make the transition from one stage of life to another in an instant, despite such legislated thresholds as ages eighteen, twenty-one, and sixty-five. It takes about twenty years to mature into an adult human; in a similar way, the aging process is gradual as our species matures and ages slowly and deliberately.

Even if shooting guns and game is not to your taste, I think you will find that the life course of the hunter offers a useful metaphor for thinking about how each of us changes over our lifetime.

It has become received wisdom among hunters that a hunter's life can be divided into five stages. The first stage is characterized by the excitability of youth. It is about shooting the gun; the focus is not on learning to aim but on the noise, the energy, the sheer thrill. A broader metaphor, perhaps, would suggest that this first stage is expansive, excited, liberating: It is about freedom. Developmentally, this equates to the hormonal exuberance of the teenage years.

The second stage is about success, which, for the hunter, means bringing home an animal. In sports, school, or even business, this stage translates to putting basic skills to use and achieving measurable results. It is a transition that many people make in college, where they settle into a routine in order to develop academically, which then carries on into the workplace.

The third stage requires more subtlety. The hunter learns tracking skills and targets a particular prey. In the larger world, the equivalent is the movement from the random to the particular, and at this stage we begin to take a more discriminating view of life and adopt goals that are more complex. Life skills, including interpersonal and workplace relations, self-discipline, and delayed gratification, grow in importance.

The fourth stage—let's call it adult maturity—involves methods, self-identified goals, and the desire to challenge oneself. In hunting it might mean using a bow instead of a gun, thereby gaining knowledge of the woods and developing greater stealth. In our lives, stage four might be equated to watching our children go off as adults while we adapt our lives anew.

As we shift into the aging years, we move to what hunters call the "philosopher stage." The goal ceases to be a moment of victory; it is not about achieving a particular goal, reaching the top of a mountain, or bagging the elusive prey we desired for years. The recollection of past triumphs becomes important; finding the opportunity to pass on hard-earned knowledge is another satisfaction. The peaks of the past have a real piquancy, but the larger joy is the sense of continuity. The horizons are wider; the focus is softer, the yearnings less acute. Safety becomes more important, as chance-taking has lost its allure.

As you think about taking charge of your aging years and working to incorporate new ideas for exercise, nutrition, and stress reduction, think about the continuum of life. I hope the philosophical you, the mellower, stage-five portion of your character, can be the foundation on which you create a sound, healthy, and appropriately disciplined regimen. It is not about instant success or gratification; it's about measured, intelligent change. It's about being happy with yourself, too.

Making the Resolution

One of the first great self-help books—it was all the rage in the Roaring Twenties—was *Self Mastery Through Conscious Autosuggestion*. The American edition appeared in the United States in 1922; its French author, Émile Coué, had trained as a pharmacist but later learned hypnotism, becoming a New Age psychotherapist well before there *was* a "New Age."

His book and method are remembered for one essential and still familiar phrase: "Every day, in every way, I am getting better and better." Coué believed that the secret to health and happiness was learning to harness the imagination. Plant the seed of self-improvement, he theorized, and improvement will come.

Scientists continue to wrestle with the mind-body connection (it exists, certainly, but its mechanisms are not so clear). But as you consider ways of lessening the impact of the passage of time during your bonus years, let's paraphrase Émile Coué. As you think about making healthy adjustments in your life, the operative assumption should be:

Every day, in every way, I am aging better and better.

Strategy Twenty-five: Take Charge of Change

You know you need to change. You probably understand the need for more than one adjustment. You need to fire up the neurons in your brain, to challenge them to expand and think harder. You may need to make different dietary choices. If your life is sedentary, there is that exercise regime you have been talking about. Too much focus on work and too little on your life? Simplify. How about enhancing your circle of contacts? Whatever the changes, you must take ownership to accomplish them.

THE ASSIGNMENT. Review the first twenty-four strategies and make a short list of the changes you need to make.

1. Divide them into categories—those you can do today, and those that will require more time.
2. Set a date each week to review progress.
3. After thirty days, review your plan.

THE RESOLUTIONS. Here are some ways to go about making changes.

- *I will do this.* That's the first resolution. You can and you will. Long-lived people tend to take charge of things, including their health and their lives.
- *I can do this.* Accepting that you can is in itself empowering. Identifying what you need to do and what you should not do is the

first step. It permits you to take the idea on board, a step in readying you to embark.

- *I will assemble a support system.* If you feel all alone, build a support system around yourself. Use your spouse or partner, peers, physician, friends, and neighbors.

- *I'll use role models.* Look for people who have achieved goals similar to those you have set. Learn from their experience.

- *I will reduce stress.* You can devise strategies that work for you to manage the stress in your life. (See *Prescription IV: Set Stress Aside,* page 103.)

- *I will find the time.* Finding the time may be a big hurdle to be overcome. Our days seem so busy that it is hard to imagine where to fit in an exercise regime, for example, or more food preparation time (because you know you can eat better at home). Even when all the time slots seem full, there are ways. Perhaps it means walking or working out at lunch. It may mean shortening your working day to accommodate shopping and cooking. How about rising a little earlier—getting up is easier now than it was when you were a teen, right?

- *I will get my eyes and ears checked.* If you haven't had a comprehensive eye exam administered by an ophthalmologist or optometrist in the last two years or your hearing checked by your doctor, do it. Good vision and hearing are important to your safety, to your ability to communicate with others, gather information, drive, and perform other life tasks. If you need glasses to correct your vision, get your prescription updated; if you have a significant hearing deficit, get a hearing aid (many health insurance plans will pay much or all of the cost).

- *I will adopt a routine.* We humans tend to be creatures of habit. If you can establish a pattern for yourself and do it for even a couple of weeks, your workouts—in the kitchen, at the gym, at your crosswords—will soon feel routine; in fact, you will probably come to miss them on the days that other obligations interfere.

- *I will avoid excess sun exposure.* Avoid direct sunlight between 10 A.M. and 4 P.M., and use a sunscreen with a sun protection factor (SPF) of 15 or higher. This will reduce your risk of skin cancer and wrinkling and age spots. Wear sunglasses when you are in bright sun. Aging eyes, because the protective pigment diminishes over the years, are more vulnerable to sun damage.

- *I will pace myself.* The best resolutions are regularly abandoned, and sometimes for quite avoidable reasons. If you set goals too high at first, then try breaking the job into parts. Healthy behaviors that are sustained over the duration of years produce maximum benefit.

- *I'll make a plan.* There is no one perfect eating regimen for all people, but there are lots of food choices, and creating menus each week can make dietary change achievable. The same is true with stress reduction: If you plan just five minutes each day for deep breathing or meditation, it can make a big difference. When it comes to exercise, the same is true: You can fit in walking or running; biking or swimming; yoga, stretching, or tai chi; hiking, cross-country skiing; gardening, raking, and other yard work; dance class; tennis or other racket sports—the list of possibilities is long. Find one or several activities you can live with and designate times each week to do them.

- *I will get enough sleep.* If you sleep less than seven hours a night and/ or wake up regularly in the night for long periods and/or have difficulty settling down, discuss your sleep deprivation with your physician. Experiment with some of the sleep strategies described in *Prescription III: Seek Essential Sleep* (see page 83).

- *I won't hesitate to amend the plan.* Change is a moving target. While early success is important and heartening, long-term maintenance is even more so. Do not be discouraged if you do not live up to your first resolutions. The profile for success involves a mixture of flexibility, humor, patience, good luck, and pluck. If parts of your plan fall by the wayside, rewrite the plan.

- *I will get the immunizations I need.* Do you have a flu shot each autumn? Have you had a tetanus booster in recent years? (See *Immunizations,* page 222.)
- *I will stretch my mental capacity.* Do you regularly exercise your brain as well your body? Work it out a little, test its endurance, build up your mental stamina. Employ puzzles, conversation, the newspaper, and any and all ways to engage your curiosity, exercise your memory, stimulate your creativity, and challenge your intelligence. (See *Prescription I: Maintain Mental Vitality,* see page 22.)
- *I will think about the upsides of aging.* They include wisdom, patience, perspective, self-knowledge, old friends, and memories. Add to this list.
- *I'll keep challenging myself.* If the games, sudoku or crosswords, become too easy, go to the next level (this is mental equivalent of the exercise cliché "No pain, no gain"). Move from checkers to chess; find a friend who loves the theater and rehearse, even memorize, a two-character scene from a play (such as *The Gin Game* or *Rosencrantz and Guildenstern Are Dead*).
- *I will reconnect.* Do you have regular contact with members of your immediate and extended family? Does your marriage need more of your caring and attention? For practical, emotional, psychological, and other reasons, a network of ties can be a safety net in the aging years. Work to weave yourself into the family skein. Social time, a friendly cell phone call from some vacation site, an e-mail birthday greeting—connections are little emotional seeds planted. (See *Prescription II: Nurture Your Relationships,* page 57.)
- *I'll try to keep a Longevity Log.* It may involve a diet diary, a record of pedometer readings, or much less quantifiable entries concern-

ing the small joys and satisfactions. This isn't about recording your failures. Keeping track is, in itself, an incentive and a reminder. Celebrate the little victories and do not sweat the setbacks. Do better tomorrow. By creating your personal behavioral database, you come to know more about what you have accomplished so you can adapt and adjust your goals for progress.

- *I will reach out.* Do you feel good about the time and energy you give to your community? Are there ways you can help others and make contact with people, both familiar and new to you? Find ways to get involved. (See *Prescription V: Connect with Your Community,* page 120.)

- *I'll roll with resistance.* When matters do not progress as you wish, use the challenges as teachable moments. You are looking for improvements; gradual is good, overnight success is rare.

- *Sometimes I'll have to shift the focus.* Some questions are not qualitative. You can weigh yourself and measure your waistline; a psychologist can assess your intelligence and a laboratory can produce a detailed report on your blood lipids. But there are deeper questions that can have health consequences, too. There are no right or wrong answers to the questions that follow, and some may seem unanswerable. But all merit your consideration and, if you think about these matters honestly, you will learn something of yourself.

1. If life is a treasure beyond measure, then have you used yours in a way that honors that gift?
2. If love is a measure of our humanity, have you given more than you received?
3. If you have possessed power in your life, have you used it to better the lives of others?
4. Has your capacity for forgiveness grown over the years?

5. Think about compassion, suffering, knowledge, the power of art, the energy of fear, the value of flexibility.

- *I will be ready to find change in odd places.* Talk with strangers. Walk in the woods. Reconnect with a distant friend or relative. Reread a book that moved you. Buy a houseplant and care for it. Go to a museum or a concert and try to let it guide you. Let your control drift.

- *If I have second thoughts . . . I'll remind myself I cannot afford to wait.* Now's the time to lose those pounds, alter those patterns, and effect healthy change. The evidence suggests that as we age, for example, exercise becomes *more* rather than less important. There is a demonstrable relationship between physical activity and quality of life. In middle age, many people fall into a sedentary lifestyle; the extra pounds and loss of muscle tone do not seem to mean much. But think about elderly friends who have trouble getting out of their chairs, or whose balance is compromised, putting them at risk of falls. Or who cannot bend over and tie their shoes. Having the strength, balance, and flexibility to go about a normal life is not something that, as the years pass, you can afford to take for granted. The same is true with exercising the brain and making friends: Find the time, make the deal with yourself, then live up to your promise.

make a contract with yourself

This is serious business, living well and living long. So let's be businesslike about setting off on your new venture. What better way than by negotiating a contract?

It does not have to be complicated, of course, but a deal is a deal.

My Longevity Contract

I, _____, the undersigned, hereby resolve to live longer by making substantive changes in my lifestyle.

Clause the First: I will depart my home on each Monday, Wednesday, and Friday at the designated time of 4:00, walk a distance that requires fifteen minutes to cover, then walk back on the same route.

Clause the Second: At no meal will I eat a portion of meat greater than 5 ounces or of cheese greater than 1½ ounces.

Clause the Third: I will attempt one crossword or sudoku puzzle each day.

Clause the Fourth: Each week I will telephone, e-mail, or contact on Facebook one friend with whom I have not spoken with in more than a year.

Clause the Fifth: When I brush my teeth each day, I will do so standing on one foot. Top teeth, left foot; bottom teeth, right foot.

Clause the Sixth: I will eat a piece of fresh, uncooked fruit with or after each meal.

Clause the Seventh: I will embrace at least one person I love every day.

Clause the Eighth: I will find a civic, faith-based, or community organization to which I will pledge three hours a month of volunteer time.

Clause the Ninth: I will abstain from alcohol on Mondays and Thursdays and restrict my intake to two drinks on any one day.

Clause the Tenth. I will make a doctor's appointment for my overdue complete physical.

Signed and Agreed _____

Date _____

This is a sample; make one that is uniquely yours and of which you can take ownership. Then go public with the contract. Share it with your spouse, your children, your best friend. They can offer you encouragement. If they scoff—they probably won't—then you have got something extra to prove, namely that they have underestimated you. Do it.

Seek Self-Efficacy

The belief that you have the capability to carry out a set of actions is called self-efficacy. If you set a goal and then accomplish it, you gain a sense of mastery. If you set a more difficult goal and reach that after sustained effort, the feeling of mastery is magnified. Self-esteem and self-efficacy are not interchangeable; the former concerns your self-worth, while the latter concerns your confidence that you can achieve a given goal.

In life, doing is believing, and a strong sense of self-efficacy can help you achieve your longevity goals. Perhaps you are aiming to improve your diet, incorporate an exercise regime into your weekly schedule, or change something fundamental about the way you live. Taking modest steps in the direction of your goal is the way to begin; small day-to-day steps will help you reach it. Your sense of well-being and confidence enhances those efforts. If you believe you can execute your plan, that sense of self-efficacy will, in the same way, help you achieve your ends.

Self-efficacy is an invaluable asset in the aging years because, in its absence, the small losses that come with age—nagging injuries, forgetfulness, the loss of a step on the tennis court—can be read as part of an inevitable decline. The risk, therefore, is resignation rather than resistance.

To bolster your sense of self-efficacy, find others like you who have accomplished what you wish to do. Modeling is no less crucial among people in the aging years than among children or young adults. Most of us learn from watching others; we gain skills and strategies from watching and talking.

Our sense of self evolves throughout life, and as we age, we need to appraise and reappraise. When it comes to physical goals, at times they need to be adapted to lessened capabilities, yet our accumulated experience and greater skills may require that changes be made. Intellectually, fewer compromises are necessary than in the physical sphere: We possess in our brains unused potentials that can be tapped with extra effort to maintain a level of function consistent with earlier years. It may take us more time to do the computation involved in solving a problem, but we probably have more corollary approaches to the problem.

If you fail to reach a goal, do not dwell on the setback. Set a new goal and try again. I find cheerleading helps, too: If you have a cohort who has been there, seek advice on structuring the next attempt. The motivation must be yours; the strategies can be borrowed.

Use your family and social assets. Ask for help when you need it, when you are looking for encouragement, advice, an exercise partner, or just someone to talk to. There are ways to reciprocate other people's kindness and generosity; this process should be generous and sharing.

Do not underestimate the qualities that come with age. We may not be stronger or quicker than our younger peers, but we've seen more. You are harder to surprise; your experience endows you with a sense of what can be done.

Don't forget that your brain is capable of changing in response to stimuli (we call it learning) and, despite myths to the contrary, the brain can rewire itself, even into old age. Some areas of the brain may be able to add new cells in response to stimulation.

Keep in mind, too, that success is not defined by your performance relative to someone else's; this is not about competition but self-improvement. If you wish to put your efforts into a context, think about them in relation to your peers, not someone much younger.

You are building something: There may be obstacles, and progress may at times be slow. Beware of allowing events you cannot control to drag you down; the sense that you are not progressing may make you vulnerable to stress and even a sense of depression. The point is not to perform like a young person; the goal is good health, a sense of joy, and a belief that longevity enables us to feel good, to do good, and enjoy our lives, family, and friends.

I told you earlier in the book that you shouldn't be thinking about this work in terms of deprivation: The goal, boldly stated, is to be happier, healthier, and more at ease with yourself. You should do something for yourself every day. Maybe it is a small food treat or spending five minutes alone. Reread a poem a day from a favorite collection, or compose one with magnets on your refrigerator. Telephone someone you care about. How about stretching out in the sun for few minutes? Play a set of tennis. Find one flower, leaf, vine, or even a craggy branch to put in a vase. Listen to a movement of music. Hum a song. Sing in the shower. Meditate.

I want you to live longer; to accomplish that I want you to do things that rouse the quiet stream of happiness that you know is there. More than anything else, that will enhance your longevity.

ACKNOWLEDGMENTS

THE *LONGEVITY PRESCRIPTION* OFFERS A WINDOW ON THE continuing work and intellectual traffic at the International Longevity Center. In addition to its staff and management, external consultants, advisers, and others who are a part of a longevity network that spans the globe, there have been hundreds, if not thousands, of experts and stakeholders associated with the center and its twelve sister centers in other countries. All played a role in developing the rich knowledge included throughout this book.

The book evolved from a staff discussion. Dr. Everette Dennis, executive director, wrote a proposal and the first draft outline. From the beginning, Megan McIntyre, former director of communications, played a vital role in connecting the substantive work of the center, along with Judith Estrine, former executive editor, who guided ILC publications from which much of this work is derived. Others whose work at the ILC helped shape the content of the book include Dr. Michael Gusmano, Dr. Kenneth Knapp, Dr. Harrison Bloom, Dr. Victor Rodwin, and Dr. Charlotte Muller. Staff members who helped coordinate efforts are Morriseen Barmore, Christine Kuehbeck, Mario Panlilio, and Milagros Marrero.

We also gratefully acknowledge members of the ILC-USA's board of directors, namely former chairman Dr. Max Link and current chair Lloyd Frank. We also appreciate the contributions of the members of the ILC's Program Advisory Group, led by Dr. George Maddox of Duke University. Seminal in the production of original reports on which some chapters are based are those who organized and led scientific consensus conferences, including Dr. S. Mitchell Harman, Dr. Michael Hewitt, Dr. Stacy Lindau, Dr. Bruce McEwen, Dr. Richard Miller, Dr. Andrew Monjan, James Nyberg, Nora O'Brien, Dr. Alan O'Connell, Dr. Marcia Ory, Dr. Richard Sprott, Dr. Michael Vitiello, Dr. Huber Warner, Dr. Phyllis Zee, and Mel Zukerman. Many of these reports were the result of collaboration with Canyon Ranch.

Finally, the ILC and Dr. Butler gratefully acknowledge the editorial and writing skills of Hugh Howard, as well as the center's literary agent, Paul Bresnick.

INDEX

ABOUT THE AUTHOR

A physician, gerontologist, psychiatrist, public servant, and Pulitzer Prize–winning author, Dr. Robert N. Butler has long been involved in a broad array of social and health matters and is known for his research on healthy aging and dementias. He was a principal investigator of one of the first interdisciplinary, comprehensive longitudinal studies of healthy community-residing older persons, conducted at the National Institute of Mental Health from 1955 to 1966, which resulted in the landmark books *Human Aging I* and *Human Aging II.* The NIMH studies found that much that is attributed to old age is rather a function of disease, socioeconomic adversity, and even personality. The research, which helped establish the fact that senility is not inevitable with aging but is instead a consequence of disease, contributed to a different vision of old age. It set the stage for the later concepts of "healthy aging," "productive aging," and "successful aging."

In 1975, Dr. Butler was selected the founding director of the National Institute on Aging of the National Institutes of Health in Bethesda, Md., where he remained until 1982. There he identified Alzheimer's disease as a major national priority. In 1982 he founded the Department of Geriatrics and Adult Development at Mount Sinai Medical Center in New York City, the first department of geriatrics in a U.S. medical school; he served as chairman and Brookdale Professor until 1995. That same year he founded and became president and CEO of the International Longevity Center (ILC-USA), a policy research and education center also in New York City, while continuing as professor of geriatrics at Mount Sinai.

Widely regarded as a leading authority on aging, Dr. Butler has served as chair of the Advisory Committee of the White House Conference on Aging (1995) and chair of the Advisory Committee of the Metropolitan Life Foundation Awards for Medical Research (beginning in 1994). He has been a consultant to the U.S. Senate Special Committee on Aging, the Commonwealth Fund, the Brookdale Foundation, the Donald W. Reynolds Foundation, and numerous other organizations.

Dr. Butler lives in New York City.

All the author's profits from this book go toward the International Longevity Center, Mailman School of Public Health, Columbia University. The ILC-USA is a not-for-profit, nonpartisan research, policy, and education organization, whose mission is to help individuals and societies address longevity and population aging in positive and productive ways, and to highlight older people's productivity and contributions to their families and society as a whole. The organization is part of a multinational research, policy, and education consortium, which includes centers in the United States, Japan, Great Britain, France, and the Dominican Republic.

Printed in the United States
by Baker & Taylor Publisher Services